Soul to Soul

Deborah Masel

Writings from Dark Places

For Sr. Carol
with love,

Debbie

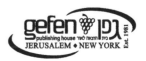
gefen
publishing house בית הוצאת גפן
JERUSALEM • NEW YORK   Est. 1981

Cover Design and Typesetting by Stephanie & Ruti Design

This project has been assisted by the Pratt Foundation
and the Australian Centre for Jewish Civilization.

To protect privacy, the names of hospitals
and of certain individuals have been changed.

3 5 7 9 8 6 4 2

Gefen Publishing House Ltd.
6 Hatzvi Street, Jerusalem 94386, Israel
972-2-538-0247
orders@gefenpublishing.com

Gefen Books
600 Broadway, Lynbrook, NY 11563, USA
1-800-477-5257
orders@gefenpublishing.com

www.gefenpublishing.com

Printed in Israel   Send for our free catalogue

ISBN: 978-965-229-559-0

Library of Congress Cataloging-in-Publication Data
Masel, Deborah.
Soul to soul : writings from dark places / Deborah Masel.
p. cm.

1. Masel, Deborah. 2. Cancer--Patients--Australia--Melbourne (Vic.)--Biography.
3. Jewish women authors--Australia--Melbourne (Vic.)--Biography. 4. Melbourne (Vic.)--Biography. I. Title.

RC265.6.M29A3 2011 • 362.196'9940092--dc23 [B] • 2011018300

For my children and my children's children

Where can I go from Your spirit?
Where can I flee from Your presence?
If I ascend to heaven You are there;
and if I descend to Hell, You are there.
And if I take the wings of the morning,
And fly to the farthest side of the sea,
even there will Your hand guide me,
and Your right hand will hold me.
And if I say, "Surely only darkness will cover me
and the light be night around me,"
even the darkness is not dark for You,
and the night shines like the day.

Psalms 139:7–11

1

My name is Deborah. I have metastatic breast cancer. Metastatic means that the primary cancer in the breast – in my case the left breast – has spread to other parts of my body: my lungs, my bones, my brain.

Please don't stop reading. I know it's scary. I'm scared too. Once I too would have closed the book. I wouldn't want to know about it. Life's scary enough, I'd say, without this. But now I'm stuck with it and I'm asking you not to shut me out.

If stories really do emerge from some fixed point, my story begins in July 2006 upon my return from a visit to Safed, an ancient Galilean city famed for its mystics, and for its melodies. My visit had been disrupted by the Second Lebanon War. Instead of studying mystic texts with fellow enthusiasts, I'd been cowering scared out of my wits in a bomb shelter, but more of that later.

The flight from Tel Aviv back to Melbourne was long enough to make the whole episode in Safed seem surreal. As I waited at the carousel for my luggage, I felt displaced and disoriented. Had I really been in Israel a week ago, when the war broke out? Had I really dodged Katyusha rockets? My suitcase, when I retrieved it, was heavy with all the books I hadn't studied in Safed.

Melbourne Airport was so ordinary, so removed from the labyrinthine cobblestoned world of Safed's old city. When I passed customs and emerged through the automatic doors, Doug, my partner, hurried to meet me. He had been anxiously awaiting my return, but after a hug and a show of relief he nodded toward a film crew waiting nearby.

"Will you speak to some reporters?" he asked.

"Sure," I said, and there they were, not one but two TV reporters, shoving mikes in my face, and there was I, waxing eloquent about my day in a bomb shelter on the Israeli side of the Lebanese border.

I was on the news that night, on two channels, and on *Lateline*. On the way home from the airport Doug told me that the crews had been waiting to interview Lebanese refugees who were traveling on my plane. Doug's mother is an Iraqi Jewess from Baghdad, and his father was born in Bulgaria. Doug is dark-haired, olive-skinned, with an aquiline nose and a moustache. You couldn't blame the reporters for thinking he was Lebanese when they approached and asked him if he was there to meet refugees. When he told them he was there to meet a refugee from the north of Israel, I got my fifteen minutes of fame.

At that time, Doug and I had been together for a mere two years, which was hard for either of us to believe. We are both very intense people. Our relationship was intense. Not stormy, just intense. We were two middle-aged divorcees trying to contend with each other's idiosyncrasies, with each other's families, with our mutual need for individual space, and for each other.

I was home from the war, and I was mildly traumatized. For a month or so, ambulance sirens set my heart palpitating, especially if they woke me and I was disoriented. Their rising and falling sounded like the whistle of a rocket before it hit the ground. As with other traumas, it seemed to pass, but was probably shoved down into the depths. No big deal. As the war escalated, I was glued to the computer waiting for news flashes. Chana, my former landlady in Safed, had stayed in the city and was sending daily bulletins. I hated feeling like the Australian tourist who'd run away. But that's what I was. I was safe at home and she was risking her life. Of course we didn't know it then, but in less than a year we'd both be facing life-threatening disease.

The war ended, unresolved, with too many Lebanese dead, rockets still falling, and Israeli soldiers still in captivity. Israel was not the country it had once been. It was no longer the valiant land of '48, nor was it the David facing Goliath of '67. The occupation was eating away at its soul. The simplicity and heroism of the early years seemed lost forever.

I resumed my life in Melbourne, and in retrospect I can see what a strange life it was.

My work as a teacher of Torah was a labor of love, I was passionate about it, and it dominated my life. When I had divorced my husband seven years earlier after fourteen rocky years of marriage, I realized that I'd need some kind of job. Not that raising three kids, running a home, and writing a few novels hadn't been work, but even more than the extra money, I wanted the respect. A self-respecting divorcée should have a job. My youngest had just started school. There really was no excuse.

I didn't have much to offer; only my writing skills. In Israel I'd been a freelance journalist. My knowledge of Torah and Jewish mysticism was still nascent; I knew what I'd gleaned from reading and from my work with the rabbi who'd turned me onto Torah, in the grossest way imaginable. Yes, I had an affair with the puffed up, manipulative little maniac who used his Hassidic stories and his Torah gems to seduce any woman who came his way. If he could net a man, he'd do that too. This was no small thing for me. It is a source of shame and disgrace. It marks a rock bottom in my life, and if I believed in a punishing God, which I don't, I believe it would justify a life cut short by cancer. I'm not speaking about adultery. I'm speaking about this particular set of circumstances. I could go into more detail, but I won't. I've excised that part of my history. The first thing I did when my cancer was confirmed was to rifle my belongings, throwing out anything associated with him, including hundreds of emails and an entire unpublished manuscript.

Shameful and difficult as it is to admit, he did introduce me to Torah. I remember the day, after months of driveling on about the great genius of the miserable manipulator by whom I'd been bewitched, my usually reticent psychiatrist threw up his hands and cried: "Don't you see? It's you! You are the teacher! Not him!"

I was shocked. Me? I? I could teach Torah?

I landed a job on the faculty of an adult Jewish education program. I still don't know how. I had no teaching qualifications and not a single day's formal Jewish education.

I didn't lie during my job interview. Paul, my interviewer, never asked me a direct question about my qualifications or experience. Some years later he told me that he went by instinct. Somehow through my discomfort and my babble he intuited that I had the makings of a good teacher.

Initially I taught one class a week, and every spare moment between those classes was spent preparing for the next. I knew a bit of fancy Kabbalah, but of the basics I knew next to nothing. I hadn't learned Judaism 101, and I hadn't practiced it. I'd been raised in a secular home. I was a fraud. Yet miraculously, my massive preparation paid off. I'd spend hours anticipating every possible question and researching the answer, and in the process I guess I stopped being a fraud. Apparently the shrink and Paul were right. I had a talent for teaching. I was popular with the students, and of course being on the faculty of such a well-known Jerusalem-based academy was qualification enough for groups and organizations who invited me to speak. The more I studied, the more I learned, but it was years before I felt at all confident in front of a class or an audience.

I studied and taught, taught and studied. I neglected my friends. I neglected my children. My priorities were stuffed. My late-night loneliness did prompt me to date a few men, with disastrous results, until one day Doug walked into one of my classes. He looked interesting, dark, and quiet. Nothing like the slightly paunchy middle-aged professional Jewish men I'd been dating.

For my classes, I usually put together a series of texts, which the students read in turns before discussing them. When Doug's turn arrived, the text was from the Book of Genesis: "It is not good for man to be alone." Doug had recently returned from Israel and seemed lost and adrift in Melbourne. I could say that we slipped into a relationship, as we would slip into a new item of clothing, but of course in relationships even a perfect fit doesn't always seem so. It took a lot of hard work. He has no children of his own, but he and my almost adult kids had to figure each other out. We didn't slip into anything. At times it was more like clearing a path in a wild jungle. It's been hard, hard work, with enough crises to make our few years together seem like fifty. Doug was an enigma to me. He wasn't like other men. He didn't need to achieve. He didn't want a "high profile" career. He followed his heart. He worked hard, and rested well. Slowly, over the years, he's shown me how to just be.

In our first year together I worked as I'd always worked, ceaselessly, stubbornly, thinking I was climbing to some kind of pinnacle, accepting every invitation to teach, to write, to perform, to do. I guess it was just another addiction. I'd worked my way through cigarettes, sex and food, and now I was into work.

In our second year together, I was tired, I thought, from trying to do it all. I was trying to parent – well, I was shopping and cooking and running a household. I wasn't parenting. I was too wrapped up in my latest addiction to be emotionally available to my children. I was trying to have a relationship, and I wasn't sleeping. I loved Doug, but I couldn't sleep with him. I'd lost the knack of sleeping with a man. All night, every night, I'd toss and turn, longing for morning. Often in the middle of the night I'd get out of bed and work in my study for an hour or so. I was worn out. I went to see a doctor, who told me I was perimenopausal. I was approaching fifty, so I guess it was the simplest explanation.

2

After the Safed adventure, I returned to work, and felt worse and worse. I started having dizzy spells when I was teaching, so I cut back some of my classes and went to another doctor. She did some blood tests, found that I was low in iron, and ordered me to eat lots of red meat.

The sleeplessness continued. I never seemed to have time or inclination to exercise. One night, after a rare visit to the local swimming pool, I had an excruciatingly painful spasm in my left chest. Doug massaged my back, and finally it passed. I figured it must have been a strained muscle, but the pain was great enough to send me back to the doctor for a full physical. Everything was in order, even my iron was fine. Right, she said. All you need now is a mammogram, and you'll be fully up to date. She left me to make the appointment with the breast-screen clinic. But of course I was busy, I was in demand, I was becoming a local celebrity. I was the woman who had beautiful words of Torah. I didn't have time.

I noticed that every so often my lungs drew in air involuntarily – something between a gasp and a sob. It was strange, but painless, and I really didn't have time to pay it too much notice.

One morning in the shower – how many lives change forever, I wonder, in the shower – I felt a huge mass in the lower half of my breast. Suddenly I had time to book a mammogram.

Doug dropped me off. The breast-screen clinic was in a picturesque neighborhood, so when I was done we planned to go for a walk. In the waiting room, I diligently filled out their multi-page information form, describing the lump in my left breast in detail. Before the scan, I showed the lump to the nurse, who agreed that it did seem rather large. The actual mammogram was excruciating. It hadn't hurt at all the last time, two years earlier. Now both my breasts, but particularly the left one, ached as they were squeezed flat between the two metal plates. They ached for days afterwards. The nurse told me that if there was anything that required further investigation, I'd be notified within two weeks. No recall after two weeks meant that everything was fine. I was free to go.

I met Doug outside, aching and a little shaken. It was a splendid day, one of those Melbourne autumn spectaculars. The neighborhood was very pretty, with many narrow side streets lined with renovated hundred-year-old homes. The gardens were unconditionally loved, not overly manicured, with beautiful weeping willows and birches. The autumn leaves were everywhere.

Doug and I love walking, not power walking, just walking arm in arm and exploring. And talking. This was a rare treat. Normally I wouldn't allow myself the luxury of this extra time in the middle of the day away from my work. I had classes to give, lectures to deliver. We were approaching a particularly busy time of year and I had much to prepare. As we strolled and chatted my sense of dis-ease lifted. Of course this was nothing! There was no breast cancer in my family and I was barely middle aged. Why, just a week ago, before I discovered the lump, I was walking our black Labrador on another brilliant autumnal day and thinking about longevity. All four of my grandparents had lived well into their eighties. One grandfather had made it into his nineties. Longevity ran in my family. I still had a lot of decades ahead of me.

My stepfather had died of cancer, an eye melanoma that metastasized to the brain. His death and the way he approached it had made a huge impact on me. I'd processed this first intimate encounter with death by writing a book about it. He was still in his sixties when he died, but of course we didn't share the same genes.

My father had died about seven years later. He had been bitten on the back of his hand by a beetle after having thrown off his mosquito net in a five-star eco-resort in Ecuador, on his way to fulfill a lifelong dream of visiting the Galapagos Islands. He developed what was thought to be flu, or possibly high-altitude sickness, and he and my stepmother cut short their trip and returned to Melbourne. As the weeks went by he became sicker and weaker. Every kind of specialist was consulted, but no one could figure out what was wrong. It could be a rare form of cancer. It could be a rare infection. We prayed for an infection. Cancer at his age didn't sound too promising, but as things turned out, it would have been preferable to the final diagnosis. He was in intensive care, at death's door before it was finally discovered that he had contracted Chagas disease, a kind of South American sleeping sickness. His was the first case diagnosed in Australia for over fifty years. It's extremely rare to find an adult with Chagas disease. South American children either die of it or survive and remain immune for the rest of their lives. The circumstances of my father's death were extraordinary enough to make it onto the evening news.

I missed both my fathers, but I guess that's another story. My story was that I came from a long line of survivors. I'm sure that if only my father hadn't been bitten by that beetle he would have lived many more years. I would live into my eighties, for sure. Maybe longer. Back then, I didn't understand the meaning of "if only."

A week passed, then another. No call came from the breast-screen people. I could relax. Or rather I could get all worked up about the important stuff again, especially about work. My first-ever real "performance" was looming. The Melbourne Jewish community's annual Israeli Independence Day celebration was the following week. This year, I was to be part of the gala event, staged for a huge audience at one of the city's largest concert halls. I had a small role in the proceedings, but a challenging one. In an interlude between major acts, I was to stand alone onstage and with the help of some barely rehearsed jazz accompaniment from the orchestra pit, recite a poem I'd written about Jerusalem. I'd wanted to read, but the director had convinced me to recite the poem from memory. Why I agreed is I suppose debatable. Maybe I was rising to a challenge, willing myself to overcome a personal limitation. Maybe I was simply ego driven. Either way, I was terrified. I recited the poem over and over, morning till night, feeling more out of sorts, exhausted, and breathless as the days passed.

When the big night arrived, I paced my dressing room, reciting and reciting, driving myself to distraction. I felt terrible. I assumed that this was what they called stage-fright, similar in nature but more intense than anything I had experienced before presenting a lecture. What if I froze onstage? What if I fumbled a line? What if I left out a whole section? What if I forgot my lines?! By the time I was called backstage I thought I'd collapse from the tension. I stood in the wings blankly watching the act before mine, employing every resource I had to keep the terror at bay. Not that I had many resources. I'd given birth three times without learning controlled breathing. My only real defense against terror was to freeze, in terror. I couldn't do that now. I had to walk onstage and recite a long poem from memory, and sound like I meant it. After all, I did write it. It was my Jerusalem.

In Jerusalem, space and time can stretch and bend,
In Jerusalem, the nexus of heaven and earth.
Jerusalem is stone and spirit, an idea, a state of mind.
Jerusalem, torn and troubled, a song of longing forever sung in a strange land.
In Jerusalem we're always looking up, for rain, for holy spirit,
And from Jerusalem we can feel God looking down, for us.
In Jerusalem, Abraham bound his beloved son,
And Jacob dreamed his ladder to the stars.
In Jerusalem, heaven and earth meet and kiss ...

Jerusalem is a Poet
Jerusalem is a Poem ...

I was having trouble breathing. Thankfully, I didn't notice the giant screen behind me that was projecting my greatly enlarged image out to the audience. I'd never done anything remotely like this before, but when I was invited to join the show, it didn't occur to me to say no. And it didn't occur to me to ask myself why I'd said yes.

The dance troupe preceding me on the program finished their bows and waltzed towards me. Clutching my mike, I walked out onto the emptied stage and placed my feet inside the floor lines I'd been shown during our one abbreviated rehearsal. I felt the spotlight on me and looked out, and saw nothing, just a few moving pinpoints of light – watches or jewels or mobile phones glinting in a great black expanse. I hadn't expected this. I forgot that the audience sat in darkness.

Looking down from Scopus through the mist
we can barely see what is
and yet we clearly see what was

tucked inside the solid shape
of what they say will be.
Across the valley, from the fog,
the future rises like a sun,
like a perfect world from an open wound,
like a promise from the breaches we have made
in our sacrificial stone.
Page falls and flutters onto page,
and God's mountain looms between the lines,
shining black on white, fire on fire,
until we see the holy Temple rise like water
from the rock where text and texture meet and merge.
And all around,
in tombs and tabernacles, minarets and spires,
in buses running scared
and empty windswept yards,
in sounds of hate and smells of fear,
the city breathes and moves
like a trembling winter bride
to the rhythms of a Heavenly Voice
calling, calling,
"I am God, I have not changed."...

I got through the performance without fumbling, walked offstage, surrendered my mike and kept walking until I found a comfortable chair to collapse into. I wanted to cry. I wanted to laugh. I felt indescribably…something. I wanted to go home. So I did, leaving my mother, Doug, and my kids in the audience to watch the end of the show.

I drove home in one great gush of relief, but my breathing was still labored. I'd had a slight cough for the past few weeks and I assumed this was the cause. Over the next week, I had to slow down considerably. I got puffed walking upstairs, teaching, and sometimes when I was just talking on the phone. The involuntary gasp had become ubiquitous. I tried to ignore my worsening condition, until it was staring me in the face. Something was very, very wrong. The barely perceptible voice that had unnerved me for weeks had now become a mighty shriek, the like of which I hadn't heard since that day in Safed when I woke to the shriek of rocket attacks on the neighboring town of Meron.

3

Late in the afternoon of that first day of the Second Lebanon War, a little less than a year before I recited my poem to all those people, I fled Safed and headed for Jerusalem. Jerusalem was the end point of a story that so closely foreshadows this story, it leads me to wonder about life, its echoes, and its travails. My journey then was not through the progressions of cancer. Then, my journey was a flight from Safed to Jerusalem, but the whole experience and the memories it triggered have returned to haunt me from the onset of my illness. I cannot ignore them. They taught me much about fear, the kind of primal fear that unhinges a person like me and makes life seem unbearable. Before I tell you the story of my journey through darkness I must tell you the story of my flight from it.

I had come to the timeless, tiny enclave of Safed, high in the hills overlooking the Sea of Galilee, to study with my long-distance teacher, Rabbi Hoffman, who had been coming to Safed from his home in Colorado every year for a couple of decades. Three days into the program, I felt as if I'd lived and learned there all my life. Three days can be a long time. My love affair with Safed was deep and passionate. Having lived in Jerusalem for a decade in my twenties, I knew the language, and I knew about falling in love. On hazy summer days, Jerusalem is a pool of liquid gold, sun on stone, ancient holy rock, synagogues, churches, mosques. Alleyways, artisans, housing complexes, shopping malls, open-air markets, and always the light, holy Jerusalem light, and air that tastes of heaven. Yes, I knew about love, and now I was deeply in love with Safed, the tiny sapphire in the Galilean hills, its stone stairways smooth with age, its cobbled courtyards echoing history.

I was lodging with Chana, in the spare room of her ground-floor apartment, in a building that was as old as the old city. There was a communal courtyard in the front, and the back looked out onto one of the many public stone stairways linking one level of this hilltop town to another.

I was away from home, away from commitment, kids, and the daily grind, and I was happy. After class on the third day of my visit, one of the students took me to visit the famous Candle Factory next to the even more famous synagogue of Rabbi Isaac Luria, the sixteenth-century kabbalist. My friend continued on to her apartment, and I was left to wander home alone. I was eating a falafel, climbing one of the old city's central stairways. I pulled out my phone and called Doug in faraway Melbourne. He told me that some Israeli soldiers had been kidnapped. I was of course disturbed, but I was not worried about myself. War and politics were far away on Doug's TV in Melbourne. I felt light and free in the sunshine that warmed Safed's ancient stones. I was having an adventure. I was forty-eight years old.

We were studying a Torah commentary called *Eish Kodesh*, in English "Holy Fire," written by the Rebbe of Piacezna in the Warsaw Ghetto during the war. Risking death, the Rebbe would preach to his congregants every Sabbath, and then after sundown, when writing was permitted by religious law, he would write his sermon from memory. The Rebbe of Piacezna was murdered in Trawniki concentration camp in 1943, but before leaving the ghetto, he buried his text, which was discovered amid the rubble after the war.

The Torah portion we were discussing begins with an account of the death of the biblical matriarch Sarah, wife of Abraham. Talmudic sages famously explained that the account of Sarah's death directly follows the account of the binding of Isaac in the text because when Sarah heard of the near-sacrifice of her only child "her soul flew from her." The sages are suggesting that Sarah died of emotional pain. A couple of millennia later, in the Warsaw Ghetto, the Rebbe of Piacezna asked a question. If the matriarch Sarah couldn't bear such pain, how much less so ordinary Jews suffering in the ghetto? We are often told that God never gives us more than we can take. No, said the Rebbe, not so. As we studied the "Holy Fire" on those few hot July mornings, I began to understand the profound compassion of this Rebbe. I had studied his text for many years, I had edited its English translation, but not until that moment had I really heard it as spoken word, as weekly sermons delivered to a beaten, bereft, suffering people. In arguing that Sarah died of emotional pain, the

Rebbe was validating the unbearable losses of his congregants. They no longer felt like failures. They were being told that it was okay to sometimes feel as if you can't go on, that you are buckling under the weight of your suffering. Even Sarah, in all her wisdom, couldn't cope.

That night, a local women's writing group gathered in Chana's living room. About six or seven women, all except me ultra-Orthodox, most with multiple children, a few tragically with none, living in cramped, old city apartments. They brought stories, beautiful stories of femininity and longing, of love and of loss, of husbands, and children, and desire.

Their stories floating in my mind, I slept well that night, and awoke before dawn to the sound of thunder, bam, bam, over and over, coming from a nearby hill. As my head cleared I heard the long whistles that preceded the booms. Through the window, I saw smoke in the distance. I leapt out of bed. Chana was in the living room. She said Hezbollah in Lebanon were hurling Katyusha rockets at neighboring Mt. Meron, aiming for an army base at the top of the hill. I didn't know it then, but the Second Lebanon War had begun.

The date was July 13, 2006, which in the Hebrew calendar was the seventeenth of Tammuz, 5766, a fast day commemorating the breach of the walls of Jerusalem by the besieging ancient Romans. Our study group arrived just after dawn, as we had planned to commemorate the fast with a pre-class visit to the grave of Habakkuk, the prophet who questioned God: "How long, O Lord, shall I cry out, and You not listen? – Shall I shout to You, 'Violence!' and You not save?" It was obvious that hostilities had broken out, but the group assured me that Safed was safe. There's nothing here, they said. Safed hasn't been touched since the War of Independence!

We drove down the hill in a convoy of two cars. I looked across the landscape and saw smoke hovering over Meron.

"Are you sure?" I asked.

"Don't worry," smiled the women of faith. "We're safe."

My sister Aviva thought otherwise. As we settled in the dawning light near the grave to learn Habakkuk's teachings, she called me from her home in Jerusalem.

"Get out!" she screamed. "They're shelling Meron! Take a bus, a taxi, anything. Pack up and leave. Head south! You're not safe there!"

My companions smiled at the over-anxious Australian tourist. My phone rang again, troubling our studies and the morning, whose silence was otherwise only disturbed by the distant sound of rocket attacks. Ashamed of my anxiety, wanting to appear unconcerned, wanting to be brave, disregarding my sister's fears, I switched off the phone.

The gravesite was desolate, and beautiful. Safed and its foothills are dotted with the graves of holy men, Safed having been the home of Rabbi Isaac Luria and his disciples. Rabbi Luria, also known as the Ari, "the Lion," formulated the theological cosmology known as "Kabbalah." Kabbalah means "reception" and refers to ideas – secrets – that have been handed down, generation by generation, from one select group to the next, throughout the centuries.

The cosmology developed by the Ari from the secrets that had come before is, oversimplified, a three-part process that bears an uncanny resemblance to Big Bang theory.

How, the Ari asks, could anything be created when God, who is everything and nothing, who always was, is and will be, occupies infinite space and eternal time? Where in the endlessness of God is there room for a creation? In order to allow for a universe, God, as it were, contracted Himself, to create within His ubiquity an empty space within which creation could happen.

God desired a world, and into the empty black hole of His desire God poured His light. This, taught the Ari, was the first act of creation, an act that is replicated in human sexuality. But in this first cosmic act the vessels designed to receive the light were not strong enough to bear it. How could anything finite, like a physical universe of time and space, contain that which is infinite and without boundaries? The vessels shattered, scattering sparks of divine light throughout the cosmos. Enter mankind. The Ari and his successors taught that the task of every human is to venture out, retrieve the sparks, and return them to their Source.

The darker the places in which we find ourselves, the holier the sparks that are waiting to be found and redeemed, because the strongest, most potent sparks had the greatest trajectory, traveling farthest, deep, deeply into darkness.

In his teachings, the Ari drew upon the wisdom of the *Zohar*, said by true believers to have been written by its main protagonist, the second-century sage Rabbi Shimon bar Yochai. Rabbi Shimon's grave is in Meron, which on that fourth morning of my visit, at the dawn of the fast day of the seventeenth of Tammuz, was copping a barrage of Katyusha rockets.

I had visited Meron and Rabbi Shimon's tomb the previous day, before joining a crowd of women in the nearby ancient stone synagogue to celebrate the circumcision of a baby boy. We women were separated by a wall from the men, and from the circumcision, but we peered through the cracks. The men were dancing and singing. The crying baby was pacified with a cloth dipped in wine. Sitting near Habakkuk's tomb, watching the smoke rise from Meron, I marveled at how much could change in such a short time. I hoped that the newly circumcised baby and his mother had found a comfortable bomb shelter.

"Don't worry," said Rabbi Hoffman, echoing his students. "Safed is safe."

After studying the writings of Habakkuk, Rabbi Hoffman waited at a distance while we women took turns to dip our bodies in the *mikveh* (ritual bath), the spring of living water, fed by an underground stream near the tomb. The water was in a small cave, difficult to access, and chilly. I emerged feeling newborn, and holy.

4

Upon our return the alleyways of Safed's old city seemed oddly quiet. We settled down in Chana's living room to resume our study of our mother Sarah's death by grief, and the teachings of the Rebbe of the Warsaw Ghetto. At midday we dispersed. Chana and I were sitting together in her living room when the first rocket hit Safed, close enough to rattle our windows.

Chana had agreed to take me in as a boarder for my few weeks in Safed. At first, she had been distant and businesslike, showing me around her strictly kosher kitchen, warning me, God forbid, against mixing the meat tea-towel with the milk tea-towel, giving me a shelf in the fridge. I found her daunting and formidable, and incredibly pious. The morning after my arrival she prayed for forty minutes, propping her prayer book on a lectern in her living room. Otherwise, she didn't speak much.

The second morning, she offered to take me to the tiny synagogue, really just a room carved into the stone, at the end of her alleyway. It was a "Carlebach" synagogue, where prayers were sung to the tune of the "singing rabbi," Shlomo Carlebach, who had brought the joys of Judaism to thousands of disenchanted young Jews in the crazy Woodstock- and dope-dominated days of the last century. Rabbi Carlebach's songs and stories had been my introduction to Judaism. Chana and I sat together in the women's section of the synagogue and swayed to the familiar tunes, prayed in whispers, and bonded. We held radically different opinions on many issues, but relations between us thawed.

Back at home, before the others arrived for the morning class, we had shared our stories. She had been raised in a secular Jewish home in Chicago, Illinois, and had remained secular throughout her marriage. Later, as a divorced mother of two in Denver, Colorado, she hadn't changed her mind regarding faith, but felt that her two daughters should nonetheless have bat mitzvahs, so on Sunday mornings she took them to classes at a nearby synagogue. She dropped them off outside the building, went to the local shopping mall, and picked them up after the class. Once, however, she needed a bathroom, so she crept into the building and made a beeline for the ladies' room, hoping to pass unnoticed by the adult class in progress in the main hall. The class was being taught by Rabbi Hoffman. Chana never stood a chance.

"Stay a while," he challenged, smiling broadly.

"No," she shook her head and hurried by. On her way back from the bathroom, he was standing in her path.

"What'll it hurt? Just five minutes."

When her girls went off to college, Chana circumnavigated the globe before settling in Safed, where she established herself as an ultra-Orthodox American divorcée who knew no modern Hebrew but many ancient prayers. Now, twelve years later, her Hebrew had improved, and she knew even more prayers. Chana was known and loved for herself and for her many good deeds by most of the residents of the old city.

When the first Katyusha rocket fell in the old city of Safed, on the morning of the seventeenth of Tammuz, I turned to jelly, and Chana became a pillar of strength.

"Sit here," she said, pulling me onto the floor. "We'll be safer on the floor."

"No, no!" I gestured wildly at the long glass panels of her sideboard, directly opposite. "We'll be covered in glass! Let's get under the table."

Chana rose to her full five foot two.

"No one but the Holy One, blessed be He, will ever make me crawl under a table," she declared, reaching for the phone.

For many years, all Israeli apartment blocks have been built with a requisite bomb shelter, but the old city of Safed had been built hundreds of years ago. There were no apartment block shelters, but there were underground rooms that had been designated as shelters scattered here and there. All the years she'd been in Safed, Chana had never had to find out exactly where they were.

"There's one a few doors from here," she said, replacing the receiver, "but it's already full. Three big families, *baruch Hashem*, and a lot of yeshivah boys."

"Chana, please! We're not comparing hotels! What does it matter? We'll sit on the floor! Let's just go!"

The air-raid sirens blared.

Chana dialed another number. "There's one on the next corner. Someone's bringing the key."

"It's locked? How can it be locked?"

"Oh, it's never been used as a shelter. It's a synagogue. Just happens to be below street level."

We heard the by now familiar whistle, gaining volume, and then the explosion, somewhere nearby. The glass in Chana's cabinet rattled.

I heard steps outside, and Rabbi Hoffman burst in. He'd been halfway back to his lodgings when the first rocket hit, and he had decided to come back to help us. Chana told him about the shelter, and we left together. Chana grabbed her prayer book, and I grabbed my mobile phone. She said she'd leave the door unlocked. Someone might need to duck in for safety.

I stood in the doorway, clutching my phone.

"C'mon, Devorah," the rabbi called in his Denver drawl. "It'll just take a few minutes."

I didn't move. Seeing the terror in my eyes, he grabbed my hand and led me out into the alleyway. Not a small gesture for one such as he, who is bound by the laws of *negiah*, which forbid him to touch any woman other than his wife.

Chana was right about the shelter. The extra few steps out in the open were worthwhile. The underground synagogue was small but relatively quiet. A group of women and a few men were sitting quietly, reciting psalms, looking for all the world as if this sort of thing happened every day. Their children sat quietly with them, or played on the floor.

Rabbi Hoffman went to the bookshelf and pulled out a volume of Talmud.

"The Piacezna Rebbe studied for years amid the terrors of the ghetto," he said. "Let's see if we can focus on a serious text for just a few minutes."

He started to read aloud. I can't remember which tractate he was reading from. The words were a meaningless blur. How could I listen to archaic arguments about archaic law? Our lives were in danger!

Rabbi Hoffman gave up. He too had failed to focus. "Then let's say psalms," he said.

I heard him, but couldn't respond. I was still frozen with fear, and in the midst of my blind terror I was reminded of one of the most moving passages in the Rebbe's book.

In early 1943, the year of the Warsaw Ghetto uprising and the subsequent complete destruction of the ghetto, the Rebbe unearthed the manuscript that he had stopped writing the previous year and carefully added a footnote. The ghetto was rubble, there was no one left. Who was he writing to? He must have believed that there would be an "after." Yet in 1943, in that terrible year of fury, he dug up his manuscript to admit despair.

In August 1941, he had written, "There are people today who make too much of the troubles, doing nothing but wasting time and words all day. Is it too much to demand that they use their spare time to learn things that do not require too much concentration, or at least recite psalms?"

In 1943, he added this footnote: "The above was written in 1941. Then – however bitter were the troubles and suffering, as is apparent from the text above – it was at least possible to lament, to find words to describe a handful of events, to worry about the survivors, and to grieve for the future…. This is no longer the case…. There exist no words to lament our woes…. There is certainly no spirit or heart left to grieve for what the future holds, or to plan reconstruction at such time as God will have mercy and save us. Only God, He will have mercy and save us in the blink of an eye."

For years, when reading this tragic footnote, I had passed over this last sentence as a figure of speech, a conventional way of ending a piece of writing. I shouldn't have. There was nothing conventional about the Rebbe of Piacezna, who in his twenties, never having left Poland or ventured outside its Jewish community, wrote a book whose English title is *Conscious Community*, which reads like a basic text of Eastern spirituality.

Years after I first read this footnote, Rabbi Hoffman brought it to my attention in a whole new way. During one of our weekly Denver–Melbourne telephone hook-ups, Rabbi Hoffman reminded me that there was nothing conventional about the Rebbe and there was nothing conventional about his times. When he wrote "God will save us in the blink of an eye," he meant it, literally. One can close one's eyes, said Rabbi Hoffman, and open them upon a whole other world. Nothing materially may change, but some inner process, some feeling of *ruach Elohim*, of God's spirit upon one, can utterly change one's perception, "in the blink of an eye."

On the seventeenth of Tammuz in the bomb shelter in Safed, I couldn't even recite psalms. My mind was paralyzed by fear. I had lived in Jerusalem in the 1980s, through the first Intifada. I had lived in fear of the "Baka stabber," who picked victims in my neighborhood at random. I had taken my firstborn to a kindergarten patrolled by armed guards and German Shepherd dogs. I was terrified of the dogs. I was once attacked by a German Shepherd. But I had never been personally attacked by some faceless "enemy." This felt like a personal attack. Rockets were being launched just a few kilometers away, with the express purpose of killing me. It was hard to believe. Paralyzing.

My mobile phone wouldn't work underground. How could I let my family in Melbourne know that I was okay? I thought of my children, of Doug, and of my mother, all in my home in Melbourne, glued to the TV. I thought of my sister in Jerusalem, frantically trying to call. And the panic surged like a missile within me.

Rabbi Hoffman was looking at me intently. "What's going on, Devorah?" He never missed the opportunity to corner a student into betraying an emotion, even here. Perhaps especially here.

"What's going on?" I croaked. "We're being *bombed*, that's what. There are missiles falling all around us and I can't even call home to say I'm all right."

"You don't feel protected down here, with us?"

"No, I don't feel protected!"

I looked at the women quietly reading psalms. They knew that God would protect them. It was as simple as that. And I knew at that moment that all my study, all my inspiring teaching, all my prayer was worth zilch. I didn't trust. I had no faith. I didn't feel protected. All my learning was academic, a sham. My Judaism was skin deep.

Rabbi Hoffman collected phone numbers and ventured up into the street to call various loved ones. He returned with Pamela, an Englishwoman who was part of our study group. Pamela and her English husband had lived in Safed for years. Her oldest daughter had recently made her a grandmother. Her youngest, Batya, was only twelve.

Batya was clinging to her mother when they entered the shelter. Pamela, a sleeping baby in her arms, sat, and Batya sat with her, silent, stuck to her mother like glue.

"She's in a bit of shock, poor darling," said Pamela, calmly, in her crisp clipped English. Apparently Batya and Pamela had been babysitting when the first missile hit Safed. They dashed out, planning to collect the baby's mother, Batya's sister, from the shop where she worked and proceed to a shelter. Batya was pushing her baby nephew in a pram. Her sister came out of the shop and was heading toward them when another missile fell, separating her from Batya, Pamela and the baby. Pamela had brought the two children into this shelter, and her older daughter, on the other side of a giant smoking crater, had gone to another.

The way Pamela told the story, it sounded like a slight mix-up at an afternoon tea party. I marveled at her composure. This must have been as new an experience for her as it was for me. Her youngest was in shock, she had no idea how and when her baby grandson and his mother would be reunited, yet she sat gracefully and calmly, one arm around her daughter, the other cradling the babe, as if this sort of thing happened all the time.

How long would I be here? I wondered, and the panic rose. I was stuck in the middle of a WAR. Why was this happening? Why wasn't I safely in my home, watching this on TV? This was not supposed to happen! Although, in a sense, according to my interminable inner script, I suppose it was. I always *knew* that disaster was just around the next bend. I always feared the worst. So why shouldn't it happen to me?

"So Devorah," said Rabbi Hoffman cheerfully. "Are you frightened?"

"Yes, I'm frightened. Of course I'm frightened. What sane person wouldn't be?" I looked around me at the women reciting their psalms, at Pamela rocking and singing to her grandson, at Batya, silently clinging, at Rabbi Hoffman grinning, and wondered, perhaps they're all mad. They can't see past their faith to the facts on the ground. We are being bombed, for God's sake! This isn't a Bible story. It's happening, here, now.

Doesn't that make it different? Not for them. But for me, then and there, it made all the difference in the world. That was other people, long ago, far away. This was ME! My children needed me. I needed me. This was not supposed to happen. And I had no faith.

It was almost evening. The fast would be broken after sunset. Pamela detached herself from Batya, handed the sleeping baby to a woman sitting nearby, and ducked upstairs for a prearranged rendezvous with Peter, her husband. He was a volunteer guard, patrolling the alleyways of the old city to make sure everyone had found a shelter. When she returned, she pulled up a chair next to me.

"You need to go now," she said, looking at me intently. "Peter's found a driver who's agreed to take you to Jerusalem."

5

Go? No, no. I can't go. It's *dangerous* out there. How could I leave the shelter? All my things, my wallet, my passport, were in Chana's apartment. All I had was my mobile phone. Drive to Jerusalem, down the side of the hill to Tiberias, out in the *open*? No!

Pamela smiled. "You'll be fine, but you have to go. It will be night soon. You're a visitor here; you should be with your family. This could go on for weeks, maybe months."

I sat stunned, bewildered. I hadn't planned on having to make such decisions.

Rabbi Hoffman smiled. "Go, Devorah. You're not coping here."

Pamela reached out, and politely took my mobile phone. Just like that. My link to the world! Crazy, really, as there was no reception in the bunker, but I thought of it as indispensable.

"Pamela, what are you doing?"

She was walking towards the stairs.

"No!" I called. "Don't take my phone!"

"Well," came the gentle reply, "you can come and get it."

I edged towards the stairs. Pamela climbed a few and waited, coaxing me with the phone. Step by step, I followed her up into the fading light, knowing full well what she was doing, and allowing myself to be taken. It was a way to side-step my fear.

Peter was waiting at the entrance to the shelter.

"Chaim will be here in a few minutes," he said. "He's got a taxi. He's agreed to take you to Jerusalem, for 500 shekels. Run to Chana's, get your things, and get back here as fast as you can."

Me? By myself? Run down the deserted alley? Through the open courtyard? To Chana's?

"You'd better go now. Chaim won't be happy if he has to wait out here."

I stopped thinking. I ran. Down the alley, through the courtyard, and into the house. I dashed to my room, swept clothes from the closet, grabbed my bag, checked that the passport was inside, and crammed everything into my suitcase. And I ran, like a wild thing, dragging the case behind me. Thank God it had wheels. Through the courtyard, up the alley. The taxi was there, engine running. Peter grabbed the case and dumped it into the boot. Pamela hugged me and threw me into the back seat, and Chaim took off.

"We'll go through the West Bank," he called out in Hebrew. "Much shorter route. We don't have enough petrol to get all the way through, but we'll get some somewhere."

If I was tense before, now I was ready to crack right open.

"Through the West Bank? Are you crazy? Nowaynowaynowaynoway. No. It's not safe!"

"We can pick up a hitchhiking soldier," he replied. "The reserves will be trying to get to their bases. There'll be a lot of them on the roads. C'mon lady. It'll be quicker and we'll be safer. They're not going to target the West Bank. If we go through Tel Aviv we could be hit."

I knew that on one level I was being unreasonable. But I so desperately wanted to feel safe. I couldn't bear the thought of driving into the night through unfamiliar territory whose inhabitants hated me.

"I can't," I said. "I won't."

He threw up his hands, then lit a cigarette, muttering something about ignorant tourists.

The radio was switched to full volume, blaring patriotic music punctuated every few minutes by breaking news. We were almost in Tiberias, at the bottom of the winding road leading down from Safed. The setting sun was behind us, and for a moment I retrieved my sense of adventure. It was beautiful, and if I was a different person altogether, I could be growing.

Chaim lit a cigarette from the stub of the last and let his window down a little.

"*Shama'at*?" He called over the blast of the radio. "Did you hear? They just hit the hospital in Safed!"

We had passed the hospital about ten minutes earlier.

"Anyone hurt?" I asked. The Hebrew newsreader was speaking too quickly for me to follow every word.

The hospital was evacuated, said Chaim. But no confirmed reports.

His mobile phone rang. I could barely hear it above the radio. He switched it onto loudspeaker. It was a woman, shrieking even more loudly than the radio. His wife, I gathered, begging him to come home.

"Soon," he said. "Are the kids home?"

"Yes, yes, come home. You should be here."

"They won't bother you there," he said. "Just sit tight."

He switched off the phone and lit another cigarette. "Where are you from?" I called.

"Nahariya."

Nahariya is roughly parallel to Safed, but on the Mediterranean coast. I could understand why Chaim's wife wanted him to come home.

The phone rang again.

"I'm going to Jerusalem, Esti," he screamed above the din. "No. Via Tel Aviv. I know, I know. What can I do? She's a tourist. She's scared. What can I do?"

Esti's raw hysteria was too guttural and hoarse for me to understand. Again, Chaim switched off the phone.

"I understand," he called back to me, consolingly. "You're a tourist. You're scared. I'll take you to Jerusalem."

Night had fallen. The fast had ended. I had neither eaten nor drunk since sunrise, all those years ago. Tiberias was behind us. The radio screamed a message.

"*Shama'at?* Did you hear that?" Chaim's ears were red. "They just hit Tiberias!"

His phone rang. His wife was begging him to come home. They were in the shelter beneath their apartment block. The kids were scared. Soon, he said, soon, and lit another cigarette.

6

Tiberias is a beautiful fishing town on the Sea of Galilee. A quarter-century ago I had been there with Jack, the man who was to become my husband. Our marriage produced three children, lasted fourteen years, and ended in divorce. Back then, before Jack and I were married, shortly after we first met, we were staying on a kibbutz near Tiberias, in a little hut close to the water. Jack was from Sydney, he was a doctor, and he spoke Yiddish. He was a "good catch." He was also wild. He took more drugs than just about anyone I'd ever known. His mother had died a few months before I met him, and his father had died a few years before that. Both were Holocaust survivors. Jack had no one else in the world; not a single living relative. He aroused my sympathy, and he satisfied my need to feel somehow closer to the great modern tragedy of our people. I'd always been attracted to James Dean–type men, but this one, a Yiddish-speaking Jewish doctor, also pleased my parents.

Our zany friends in Jerusalem had given us a tab of acid to bring with us, a little square of blotting paper soaked in LSD. Jack put half on his tongue, half on mine. It was August, unbearably hot. We waded in, sinking into the water that should have been walked upon. He mistook himself for a fish. I mistook my handbag for a baby, and worried that it was becoming overheated in the hut. After an hour, or maybe the next day, we drove to Tiberias, to eat. He drove too fast, and I was scared. All my life, nothing, no dream, no drug has ever succeeded in quenching my fear for long. My fear was primal, omnipresent, an irresistible force waiting to meet an immovable object. Immovable, incurable cancer.

In Tiberias we sat by the water and ate hot chips. I watched the passing parade.

Everyone in town had a disability: distorted faces, useless limbs, twisted feet. Jack fed a mangy half-bald dog. Later, we went to a fancy outdoor restaurant, overlooking the Sea of Galilee, and ate St. Peter's fish. Came time to pay, and we had neither cash nor credit card. All left in the hut. Fear, more fear. We'll be arrested! We'll have to work in the kitchen all night! I approached the desk alone.

"Come back tomorrow," said the proprietor, "and fix us up."

I returned to our table, triumphant. The man who is now my ex-husband was standing by the water, surrounded by diners at their outdoor tables, pissing into the Sea of Galilee.

Now the seaside restaurants in Tiberias would be empty. Everyone would be underground, waiting for another Katyusha.

"I'm going to stop soon to get petrol," Chaim called over his shoulder. Tiberias was behind us and the sky was full of stars. The first three signaled the end of the fast. I clutched my handbag, ready to jump out at the petrol stop to buy food and drink.

The music was interrupted by more breaking news.

"*Shama'at?*" Chaim shouted. "Did you hear? Tiberias!" He indicated, and pulled into the petrol station. I bought Coke and chocolate bars for myself, and for Chaim. As he stood outside the taxi, filling the tank, his mobile phone rang again. He ignored it, and kept filling. Hurry, was all I could think. Hurry, take me away from here.

This was crazy, I'd come for a quiet study retreat, and I was running for my life. I felt like a rabbit caught in high beams. What was it about me and drama? I'd never been on a roller coaster in my life. I understood the fear, but I could never fathom the thrill. I didn't want fear. I didn't want drama. I liked the merry-go-round. I liked certainty. Why was this happening to me? Was this normal? Were all lives as crazy as mine?

When I was six I was run over by a car. My father had taken me to the park. My mother was with her lover. My father and I, holding hands, had crossed the road. We were safely on the pavement when we heard a car swerve. It had missed the turn into the side street, and was heading for the pavement, where we stood. My father, seeing the out-of-control vehicle's trajectory, pushed me to the ground, and the car went over my prone body, wheels either side of me. I remember lying under the car. I remember being pulled out from under, shocked, bruised, but basically, miraculously unharmed.

Years later my mother told me I wet my bed that night. I remember being under the car. It's one of my earliest memories. Mostly, my early childhood is a blur. But I remember being under the car. I remember the dark, the fear, the wheels either side of me, wheels that might have crushed my body, left me paralyzed, or dead. I remember the smell of grease and petrol, and the growing number of ankles and feet, milling by the car. Women's stockinged ankles, a workman's tough boots. I remember being dragged out by my legs, by a passerby. My father was frozen in fear. Being under the car was like being in the bomb shelter. It was like being a cancer patient, waiting for test results. I remember it well, because it seemed to me that I was there for a long, long time.

We were heading for Tel Aviv. Chaim was driving fast. The radio was blaring, and I was devouring Coke and chocolate.

"Oy! Nahariya's hit!" Chaim's home town. This time Chaim called his wife.

"Yes," she said, "we're all okay. We're in the shelter. The kids are scared. Come home."

"Okay," he said, "okay. I'll call you back."

"I'm going to call around," he shouted back at me. "I'll find someone else going to Jerusalem and transfer you. I have to get home."

"Yes, yes, of course."

The closer we got to Jerusalem, the safer I felt. Safe enough to feel sorry for Chaim's wife and kids.

I laughed hollowly, amused at the thought of Jerusalem as a safe haven. I had lived in Jerusalem throughout the first Intifada, when the "city of peace" was considered one of the most dangerous places in the country, or, for that matter, in the world. Terrorist attacks were rife. For years, we were advised to get down on our hands and knees and peer under our cars before we drove off, to make sure no one had planted a bomb there. We were all – Jews and Arabs – stressed and tense. In the '70s and early '80s, there had of course been tension, but I had felt safe enough, even in Arab East Jerusalem. Before the Intifada I often visited the Muslim quarter of the Old City. Our favorite café, with the best Turkish coffee in the city, was just inside the Damascus Gate. We often drove to Jericho and to the Arab village of Abu Gosh to eat humus that was hands down better than anything we could get on our side of town. At least once a week I took my small son to Jaffa Gate to buy fresh pita bread from Arab vendors. I had been a welcome guest in the home of a Palestinian businessman who had been treated by Jack in Jerusalem's Shaare Zedek Hospital.

With the Intifada, all that ended. Unless "crossing over" was unavoidable, we stuck to our side of town, and they to theirs. And then, in 1991, came the war – the first Gulf War – and I took my two kids and fled. Jack, an army reservist, had been called up. My four-year-old son and I had been issued gas masks, his child-sized, and I'd been given a kind of tiny oxygen tent for my eighteen-month-old daughter. In the event of a chemical attack, I'd have to fit myself and my son with masks, and place the baby in the plastic tent and feed in oxygen through a tube.

This was not my idea of fun, nor did I see it as a life adventure. I loved Jerusalem, passionately. I loved its glow, its special scents and stones and skies and valleys. As the child of inveterate travelers, I had grown up on four continents. I had seen magnificence, and beauty. But only with Jerusalem, the jewel in the crown of a tired and troubled land, was I in love. I just didn't love the danger. Can one have one without the other? Can I imagine a Jerusalem of quiet sleepy suburbs, placid inhabitants, gentle descents into night? Would Jerusalem be Jerusalem without the fire in its belly, without the strife?

I'd booked flights to Melbourne for myself and my children a few months earlier. I had been planning to take the kids for a three-week visit to see my father, who had never met my baby daughter.

A few weeks before we were due to leave, Jack's army reserve unit was called up. He'd hardly been home since then. With war imminent, and many people, mostly tourists, scrambling to leave, I was very grateful for the pre-booked tickets, although I wasn't happy about the route, through Cairo. It had seemed like a good idea at the time – peace time – much cheaper than the direct flight to Bangkok. Before we left I cut all the Hebrew labels off our clothes. I told my son not to speak Hebrew, only English. We were Australian. We had Australian passports.

I felt like a coward, and in the eyes of many Israelis, I was. It was a matter of pride, and most probably national survival, to carry on during a war as if nothing was happening, only more so. People would tell jokes about Saddam and swing their gas-mask boxes as if they were fashion accessories. The less fearful, the more highly they were regarded.

To Australians born and bred, taking young children out of a war zone probably seems the logical, responsible thing to do. But we Jews, amongst others, often have a different perspective. War zones are part of the recent history of most of our families. We are raised to regard Israel as the only true haven, and many of us choose to live there, at least for periods of our lives. Within my community, my having lived in Israel for ten years is not so extraordinary.

7

Chaim had reached a friend who was also driving his taxi on the road from Tel Aviv to Jerusalem. They arranged to meet at a pit stop, where I would transfer cars.

"I'd better pay you," I said, reaching for my purse. "Mastercard?"

"I can't take cards," said Chaim. "Only cash."

Chaim's taxi was most probably fitted with credit-card facilities. I realized that this very special journey from Safed to Jerusalem, with its special price, was on his own time. This had to be a cash deal, under the counter.

"I don't have any cash."

All I could think of was to call ahead to my sister and ask her to bring cash when she came to meet me at the entrance to Jerusalem. But that would mean that Chaim would have to take me all the way.

Since I fled Israel in 1991, the gap between rich and poor had widened considerably. The rich were getting richer and the soup kitchens were multiplying. Chaim was probably extremely grateful for the opportunity to make some extra cash on the side, despite the danger and his wife's pleadings.

He called his friend and cancelled the rendezvous.

"Stick with me," he called to the back seat. "We're nearly there anyway. I'll take you to Jerusalem."

We had begun the familiar ascent to Jerusalem. The roadside was littered with the rusty remains of primitive tanks, left as a memorial to those who fought in the War of Independence, when a ragtag army of farmers and Holocaust survivors, armed with anything they could steal, beg or borrow, had triumphed against overwhelming odds. With independence, Jerusalem was divided, and one of the oldest cities in the world continued one of the longest histories of violence and dispute.

We were going up to Jerusalem! My heart beat faster. Although it was night, I knew the road well enough to picture it all – the timeless view, the hairpin bends, the entrance to the city, and a little further, the central bus station and Binyanei Ha'uma, the famous convention center. We were to meet my sister in the parking lot in front of the center.

My half-sister Aviva is twelve years my junior. As an infant she had regarded me as another parent. And I had loved her as a baby and as a little girl, with parental, unconditional love. As adults we had struggled for years to redefine our relationship. But this was a moment when no definitions were necessary. She leapt out of her car, into my arms.

"Thank God you're safe!" Tears were streaming down her face. "Thank God, thank God."

Aviva is shorter and slimmer than I, and for a moment she clutched me the way a child clutches her mother.

Aviva gave Chaim the cash, and he wished us well. He hesitated. I could see he was wondering if I was too observant to accept a hug. I held out my arms and he laughed as we embraced.

"Have a safe journey home, Chaim."

"No worries," he said. "I'll be there in no time." I wondered if he was planning to return through the West Bank.

My sister took me back to her apartment on the outskirts of Jerusalem. We watched a few news bulletins with her husband, Gil, to ascertain that the war really was in full swing, and I went to bed, in the spare room.

I don't know when I've ever felt so safe. This was like being pulled out from under the car, or like arriving at the farmhouse the time my mother nearly drove us off a cliff and had to walk us down a mountain, at night, in Malaysia.

My brother and I were spending the summer with my mother and her new husband in

Singapore. We had driven from there to the Cameron Highlands in Malaysia where David, my stepfather, was attending a conference on tropical medicine. Late one afternoon, while he was at the conference, our mother decided to take us to the peak of a nearby mountain, to see the sunset.

The road to the top was steep, with one hairpin bend after the other, each sharper than the one before. Our wide American car didn't take the turns too well. There was no railing on the edge of the road, just a very steep slope to the bottom of the mountain. No way back, either, until we got to the top, as the road was too narrow for a U-turn. When we were near the top the car didn't quite make the bend. Our mother stopped the car at the very edge of the precipice and pulled on the handbrake. She'd need to reverse to get back on the road, but when she released the handbrake the car would go over the cliff if she didn't reverse quickly enough. So she did something I've never quite been able to fathom. I must have been about eight and my brother would have been about ten.

Our mother told us to get out and wait by the side of the road, even though there was no side, just a narrow road on which cars and motorbikes could come around the bend from either direction. We were to wait while she tried to get the car back on track. Night was falling. We were miles from anywhere, and mobile phones would not be invented for another thirty years. I guess she must have noticed the gaps in her logic, because, after starting the engine, she turned it off again, abandoned the car at the edge of the precipice, and taking our hands started to walk us down the mountain.

The sky was inky by then and we could hear bird shrieks and animal sounds coming out of the darkness. The previous year, an American had mysteriously disappeared in these parts, presumably eaten by tigers. Our mother must have heard about this, but nevertheless she really rose to the occasion. We could feel her terror through her trembling hands, but she tried to pretend we were having fun.

"Let's sing," she said. "Let's sing 'The Sound of Music.'"

Even at the time, as we were walking down the mountain, I could picture us, a mother and two children edging down a steep slope at night, terrified by the thought of animal attack, singing "The hills are alive…" Quite the Family von Trapp, or their very dark shadows.

The terrain changed. We were passing through some kind of sloping field, perhaps a tea plantation. When we sighted electric lights glowing in a farmhouse ahead we broke into a run. Soon we were safely inside, drinking hot tea, covered in blankets. Our hotel was called and my stepfather notified. The elderly couple who lived in the farmhouse were very kind. I had the feeling that they had entertained crazy Western visitors like us before.

Curled up in my sister's spare bed after my dramatic taxi ride to Jerusalem, I felt as I had in that farmhouse. I was inside, warm and dry, and all the wildness was out there, neatly packaged for my convenience on a TV screen, where it should be.

For another ten days I wandered the streets of my beloved Jerusalem, touching the familiar stone and marveling at the changes – a freeway cutting right across the city, giant shopping malls, luxurious suburbs, and ever-growing slums. I visited Machane Yehuda, the great sprawling market near the city center.

A quarter of a century ago, Jack and I had lived here, in an apartment directly opposite the entrance to the *shuk*, the market, when we were first married. The *shuk* was largely unchanged; it still reminded me of a living, breathing organism, flooded with color and noise and aromas. Fruit stalls, butchers, spice stalls, cheap clothes, vendors calling out their wares, round women with kerchiefs on their heads, haggling, bargaining. I remembered the weirdness to which I could never quite accustom myself as I watched in the evenings through my apartment window while the *shuk* shut down, like a giant beast lowering itself onto its knees to sleep, or pray. The sounds of stalls slammed shut and locked, people emptying onto the street, and later, late at night, men with massive hoses watering away the filth, preparing the *shuk* for its 5 a.m. start the following day.

I loved the market and I loved Nachlaot, the ancient neighborhood of cubbyhole shops and tiny synagogues and squares that sat adjacent to it, but I feared them also. Fear, my fellow, my life-companion. In these streets, for three years, I had been stalked.

Before I married Jack, I had lived in Nachlaot, in an old, stone, two-story building that had been divided into four one-room flats. My room was my entire home. It looked out onto the narrow cobbled Nachlaot street, filled with other old buildings just like ours, with washing hanging from lines suspended between windows, with sounds of laughter and tears, distant sounds from the *shuk* and the Old City, and sounds of children playing in the street below. I felt very cool in that flat, like the best kind of Jerusalemite, the kind that loved the city down to the dirt in the pavement, down to the soles of her feet.

The window of my little stone apartment was covered with a silky curtain, opaque enough to blur the view but still let in the light. Or so I thought. Years later, after I had married and moved, I learned that Eli, who lived across the street, loved looking through my window when I was dressing, and especially when I was wandering around naked after a shower. Eli was a short man, and his hunched back made him even shorter. One of his legs was shorter than the other, so he walked with a severe limp. Eli had some kind of skin virus, and his face was pocked with greenish dots.

He was always out in the street, smoking. I felt sorry for the poor guy and said "shalom" to him whenever I passed by. He would beam and return the greeting. Sometimes he tried to engage me in longer conversations, but I'd say a few polite words and move on. I didn't know he was watching me through the window. I didn't know he'd become obsessed. I didn't know that he believed I was his wife from a previous incarnation, and that sometimes he believed I was his sister. I didn't know until I married and moved to the apartment opposite the *shuk* and found Eli smoking outside on the street, all day, every day. He followed me. He sat on the step by the security door of my apartment block. He terrified me.

I told the police. They already knew him. They had words with him. He kept following me. Once he gained access to the building and I returned from shopping to find him standing on the landing outside my door. He smiled at me and tried to tell me about us, about him and me, as I jiggled my baby on my hip and fumbled with my key. Jack was home. He came out onto the landing, pinned Eli against the wall, punched him in the nose, and literally kicked him down six flights of stairs. I was shaking from fear of Eli, from terror of violence. Eli never came into the building again, but he kept following me. I started getting phone calls. Deep breathing. The police picked him up again for twenty-four hours. They couldn't keep him longer, they said, or charge him unless I accused him of physical assault.

I felt trapped, stuck under the car with no way out. More anonymous phone calls. He followed me through the *shuk*, every day. I feared for my child. I went to police headquarters, a magnificent building in the Russian Compound.

"Okay," I lied. "He grabbed me, tried to violate me, but I got away."

Eli was arrested. He got six months. Six glorious stalk-free months. As soon as he was back on the streets he was back at his station outside my building. Nothing can stand in the path of true love.

"You're my wife," he pleaded, as I fumbled with the key, looking away. "You're my sister."

We moved to Nayyot, a peaceful suburb of beautiful homes built by wealthy Anglo immigrants to Israel. After Nachlaot it was a lovely change. No dirt. No noise. I shopped in an air-conditioned supermarket and didn't venture near my beloved *shuk* or even to Nachlaot for over a year. I never saw Eli again. I don't know what happened to him.

During those few days in Jerusalem after my flight from Safed, I re-experienced the unifying buzz of love and brotherhood that goes hand in hand with a national emergency. Those in the south of the country opened their doors to the thousands of refugees streaming out of the north. As the army reserves were called up and the young Israelis in the midst of their compulsory army service were sent into Lebanon, parents and spouses all over the country became personally and terrifyingly involved. I met with a number of refugees from Safed and stayed in phone contact with those brave souls who'd decided to stay in their homes in the north. And I began to think about the war. I knew that most of the rest of the world saw Israel as the aggressor; I hated what was in the cards for so many Lebanese civilians, but I had been in Safed when the rockets fell, I had seen the faces of the families of the kidnapped soldiers. I craved simple solutions. I wanted an absolute faith in right and wrong in a world where everything was blurred.

When it was time to leave, my sister drove me to the airport. As I sat, finally alone in the departure lounge, I reflected on the past few weeks. I'd come to Israel, to Safed, anticipating a period of intense study. I'd been looking forward to living amongst strangers, and during those first few peaceful days I'd fallen wildly in love with the tiny old city of Safed. Then, chaos. Fear from the sky, sirens, running in the streets, hiding in shelters, fleeing to Jerusalem. A totally other experience.

But isn't this almost always the case? I cross the road, holding my father's hand, arrive safely at the pavement, and wind up under a car. I set out with my mother to admire a view and wind up groping in the dark to the shrieks of wild Malaysian animals. I thought I was safe in my little self-contained room in Nachlaot, but I was actually exposed to a madman who stalked me for years. What is it with me? Do I secretly crave this stuff? Do I subliminally seek it out? But I'm too scared to go on a roller coaster!

8

After my Safed adventure, I returned to Australia relieved to have escaped, yet again. In my nearly fifty years on this planet I had come to believe that for cowards like me there was always a way out, a way around the fear. No matter what sort of mess I got myself into, someone would save me. I was about to learn otherwise.

A few days after I recited the poem about Jerusalem at the Independence Day celebrations, I was on the phone with Rabbi Hoffman for our weekly class. For years, on and off, we'd studied *Eish Kodesh*, the text we'd been learning as a group in Safed the previous year. There's nothing in the world quite like this text. Before the war, the Rebbe of Piacezna had spent years contemplating the principle of God's ubiquity, theoretically and experientially. In a diary he kept before the war, he wrote of his desire to know that he was always in God's presence, even in the valley of the shadow of death. "My soul takes courage," he writes. "Even in the depths of hell I shall not fear, for You are with me!" His early theoretical writings explore the concept of darkness as a source of light, of God's hiddenness as the source of human enlightenment and revelation. Darkness, he argued, the sense of exile and separation, gives rise to a longing in the human heart, a yearning to connect, which we call spirituality. It is the very sense of separation that is the basis of revelation.

These beliefs made him particularly well equipped to confront the great darkness of the Holocaust. The deeper the darkness became, the greater his spiritual response. I once heard a greatly respected scholar and mystic say that in his opinion, the Rebbe of Piacezna experienced revelation at the level of prophecy in the final months of his life.

I can't remember which particular teaching from the *Eish Kodesh* Rabbi Hoffman and I were studying that Friday morning, but I do remember hearing my mobile phone ring in the kitchen, and I remember hearing Doug answer it. I remember trying to read the passage we were studying aloud over the phone, as was our custom, and I remember asking Rabbi Hoffman to take over, because I was out of breath. After studying, we chatted for a few minutes before ending the call. This I remember very, very well. Rabbi Hoffman reminded me that in a few more months he'd be returning to Safed for his annual teaching round.

"Why don't you come too, Devorah," he asked. "Perhaps there'll be another attack," he chuckled, "and you'll get to sit in the shelter again, and this time maybe you won't panic. You could have a second chance, an opportunity to redeem yourself."

He was joking, but as with all his jokes, he cut straight to the quick. I had panicked in the shelter, and I had run away. Given another chance to experience that degree of fear, would I panic again, or could I possibly put what we had been learning from the Rebbe of Piacezna into practice?

The call Doug had answered on my mobile phone had been from the breast-screen clinic. Could I come next Tuesday to their center at a nearby hospital for further tests? Something turned in the pit of my stomach, like some kind of sleeping monster awakening. My bowels turned to water. I had to run to the bathroom. I knew. In the pit of my stomach, I knew everything. I knew what wouldn't be verified for another four weeks. I knew with a knowing I'd never known before. I knew with all my trembling being.

It seemed hugely difficult to clear a whole day in my busy calendar. Back then I thought that more than one medical appointment per year was unreasonably excessive and an unfair demand on my time.

In the interim, I had to get through the weekend. I tried to stay busy and not think too much, but the anxiety pushed through most of the time. I was becoming more and more breathless. On Sunday I attended a meeting of my spiritual community. I'd been a member of this community since its rather ignominious inception, ten years earlier. We'd started out as a rather shady cult-like group gathered around the aforementioned twisted rabbi, who, it must be admitted, knew how to turn people onto Torah.

He traumatized us enough to render us radically opposed to central leadership. We've been a rabbi-less congregation ever since. But we are learned. We run our own services and promote the ultimate in women's participation within an Orthodox framework. We like to think of ourselves as cutting edge, as radical. And once a year or so, the inner circle gets together to argue about where we're heading. The meeting was at a building in the university, on the fourth floor. I arrived together with Andrew, who happens to be a radio-oncologist. There's no shortage of brains in our congregation.

"Let's take the stairs," he said.

I looked at him and balked. "I can't," I replied. "I'll get too out of breath. I think I have some sort of chest infection."

He looked at me. "A woman your age ought to be able to climb stairs," he said.

I took the lift, and tried to focus on the meeting. But my mind was elsewhere. Before we finished, I leaned across to Andrew and asked if I could speak with him privately before he went home. After the others left, we sat alone at a big round table, and I told him the story so far. Andrew is a gentle soul, a lover of music, softly spoken.

"Well," he said, "you don't need to panic. Many women are called back and most are fine. You could have a cyst. Let's just wait and see."

He seemed worried. He wasn't reflecting my concern. I saw something in his eyes that knew more than he was saying.

Doug and I were among the first to arrive at the clinic on Tuesday morning. I'd brought some books with me to read in preparation for a talk I was due to give the following week. My workaholism was a great bone of contention between Doug and me. Looking back, I think it was threatening to ruin our relationship. Doug is a very sensitive, very intelligent man who seems to have no desire to achieve for achievement's sake. Childless from his previous marriage, he is financially independent, and frugal enough to be able to spend his time as he pleases. If a project captures his imagination, he gives it everything, and more. Between projects, he is content to cultivate our garden, and sit for hours in it, smoking cigarettes and staring at the lily pond.

It's not that I don't understand such a life. I find it appealing, and I even remember it vaguely. It's just that since becoming a mother of three with enough financial support but next to no physical or emotional help from husband and parents, I've had to amputate that part of myself. Quiet, reflective time disappeared abruptly with the first child, and life became more and more about fitting as much as possible into little time. Like many women, I was a mistress of multitasking and a wizard at being everywhere at once, which meant that I was never completely anywhere. Sometimes I'd look out of my study window to the quiet garden where Doug was sitting, and feel alternately wistful, worried, and resentful. Had I made a mistake? He wasn't like other men in our community. He was super-sensitive, and strikingly honest about his feelings. But I wasn't partial to other men in our community. I didn't much like their drive, their business, their assumed superiority. I loved Doug. We'd had truly wonderful times together, just walking, or driving to the hills for a day or two. We talked and talked. It sounds corny, I know, but he was my best friend.

So in the waiting room I read my books and made notes, and Doug sat motionless, staring mildly into middle distance. I was taken to a cubicle, told to strip to the waist and given a hospital gown to wear. More women arrived. Soon the waiting room was crowded with bra-less green-gowned women, most with friends or partners, flicking through magazines and trying not to worry.

One by one, we were called inside for a mammogram. This time, they only scanned my left breast. Back to the waiting room. When all the mammograms were finished about half the women were told they were free to leave. They left smiling, savoring the sweetness of relief. The rest of us watched silently, envying them. Then we were called one by one, for a breast ultrasound. My poor left breast was already tender and sore, but I gritted my teeth. The day was fast becoming surreal. I felt as if I was moving without motion, like in a dream, from one moment to the next.

The technician poked and prodded at my breast and recorded the measurements that appeared on her computer screen. As the morning progressed, I was withdrawing into my shell, feeling more and more passive. It seemed that it wasn't taking long for me to become the ideal patient.

Back to the waiting room to hold hands with Doug and wait for the next verdict. I'd lost interest in my books, and it seemed somehow frivolous and perhaps bad karma to pick up one of the trashy magazines from the table. I sipped cold water from a polystyrene cup and waited. I was a patient, so I was trying to be patient. More women were sent home. There were only three of us left. The doomed. A nurse came out and sat with Doug and me to explain that I would be having a biopsy, well, a couple of biopsies. It seemed that there were two lumps in my breast. It wasn't a complicated procedure.

Samples of the lumps would be suctioned out of the breast through a needle and sent for analysis. Hours ago the thought of this would have horrified me, but by now I was quite numb. I nodded mutely and awaited my turn.

I was led back to the room where I'd had the ultrasound and laid out on the bed. I opened my hospital gown and out flopped the offending breast. It looked like a sacrificial offering, waiting there on the operating table. In came the doctor.

"Oh," she said, approaching the bed. "Do you remember me?"

No, I didn't, but I smiled, wanting to please. She was about my age, blond, Anglo-Saxon, could have been school captain of a private ladies' college a number of decades ago. I didn't recognize her at all.

"I'm Elizabeth's mother," she said, "from primary school."

I pondered. Ah! Elizabeth! When my kids had been in primary school I'd volunteered to teach a creative writing class for gifted sixth graders. Elizabeth had been one of the most gifted of all.

What a relief to know that the woman who was about to stick needles into my breast was an old friend. I looked at her name tag. Sue. She smiled and said she was sorry we had to meet again here. Not as sorry as I was, I responded. She chortled. Elizabeth had loved my creative writing classes, she said. Elizabeth was at uni now, studying medicine. I wondered if she still wrote short stories.

I relaxed. I was in good hands. I don't remember the biopsies as being particularly painful. I suppose she used local anesthetic. In the end she took three of them, as another suspicious area was picked up elsewhere on the same breast. The nurse bandaged it up and told me not to lift or raise my arms for a few days.

It was mid-afternoon by the time I put my bra and shirt back on. We were told to return first thing Friday morning for the results.

Wednesday. Thursday. Friday. Those two and a half days still seem interminably longer than the two and a half years that have elapsed since.

We decided to tell no one, as nothing had been confirmed. I told the kids and my mother that I'd bruised my shoulder and had to be careful not to knock it or strain it. My mother had that same worried look in her eyes.

At night I lay in bed next to Doug and worried. In her book on Genesis, my mentor,

Avivah Zornberg, had written that worrying originally meant attacking, tearing limb from limb, and it still means working away at something, trying to pull it to pieces. That's how they felt, the thoughts, the fears, worrying away at my peace of mind. I hardly slept. I felt as if I'd hardly slept for years. And that was probably true. As a child and teenager I'd needed a lot of sleep. If I didn't get at least eight hours I could barely function the next day. I guess I just didn't have the right constitution.

All that changed of course after the birth of my first child. A full night's sleep became a thing of the past. Despite being heckled and pushed by Israeli friends and neighbors to let the baby cry himself to sleep, I just couldn't do it. I ran to him every time he called, two, three, seven times a night. I walked up and down, up and down at 3 a.m. with him on my shoulder, looking down through the window at the sleeping *shuk*, until he fell asleep. Then I'd creep back with him to the cot and ever so gently lay him down, but often he woke and screamed, so I'd pick him up again, and walk up and down, up and down, humming, wanting to out-scream him. I did the same for my second child, and for my third. Jack didn't help all that much. He had to work, sometimes up to seventy-two hours in the hospital emergency room without coming home for a break. By the time the kids were all sleeping through the night, when we were back in Australia, I'd lost the capacity to sleep. I was discovering Torah and Jack was riding a Harley-Davidson. I was learning Sabbath observance and he became the official doctor of the Hell's Angels. I was mooning over a moon-faced rabbi and he was drinking in topless bars.

After I turned to Torah, my growing estrangement from Jack kept me up later and later, in the hope of creeping into bed after he'd fallen asleep. And when I did finally get there, my head would buzz with thoughts, with snippets of songs replaying over and over, and with worries. I'd finally fall into a fitful sleep, only to wake an hour or so later. I couldn't seem to relearn how to sleep the way I had in my youth.

It wasn't Jack's fault. I was the one who had changed. When we met, I had not yet let go of my adolescent wildness. After a timid and often terrifying childhood, my behavior swung to the other extreme a year or so after I joined my mother and stepfather in London. My brother had failed to adapt to life in London, and had rejoined our father and his new wife in Melbourne. My mother hated the London winters. She and my stepfather took to avoiding the worst of it by returning with my baby half-sister Aviva to Australia when London was at its blusteriest. They were slowly making a fortune on the Melbourne property market. I was boarded out with the families of girlfriends.

The first time they left me in London, in my first year of high school, I stayed with Susan Round and her family. Working class, they lived on the top floor – formerly the servants' quarters – of one of those old English multi-story stately homes, most of which have been converted into blocks of flats. My parents had paid well for my board, so Susan's mother insisted on serving me a cooked breakfast every morning – sausages, bacon, eggs, toast. Dinner, or supper as they called it, was fairly similar. At school, for what I called "lunch," we had LSD, London School Dinners, invariably meat and potatoes followed by pudding. Nonetheless, I was a skinny thing when I began my stay at the Rounds', and barely a shadow when I left. In that attic flat I experienced terror as never before.

The terror visited me in the form of a television series. The Rounds watched telly most nights after supper, and I watched with them. On Sunday nights we watched a BBC series called *Six Wicked Women*, one for each week of my stay. Every Sunday I was subjected to women who imprisoned, who tortured, who dismembered, who brutalized, who drove to insanity. Susan and I shared a bed, as there wasn't a separate one for me. The wicked women series had damaged my soul. I was ashamed of my terror and my weakness. I told no one. I sat in front of the telly with the others, then lay rigid, wide awake in bed all night, every night, terrified of my thoughts, terrified of the images behind my eyes, terrified of waking Susan. By the time my parents came to take me home, I had huge black shadows under my eyes. I never told them why. I was too ashamed.

My second boarding-out experience was quite different. This time I stayed with Mandy Darville, the only child of a divorced, generally out-of-work actress who drank in the afternoons and chain-smoked. I liked her. She was easygoing and she treated me as an equal. Mandy and her mother lived in a basement flat in Notting Hill Gate. At night Mandy's mother would go out, or entertain in her bedroom, and Mandy and I would crawl through her bedroom window, climb up onto the street, and head for Portobello Road, and a bit of fun. We were both fourteen, tall, dark-skinned, big-eyed and skinny and we were beginning to realize that in the eyes of others, that wasn't such a bad combo. I can't remember doing anything dreadful on those nights out. We wandered around, talked to strangers. We learned how to smoke. I got to sip a few drinks. We were lucky. The strangers we met were street people, but good people. Like many adolescents, I felt as if I had stepped right through my childhood terrors and shattered them, as if they were panes of glass.

Six months later, I was an addicted smoker. I hung out with a bad crowd at school. We regularly wagged (cut class), even though we often had nothing better to do than board a Central Line train with a ticket good for one stop and go round and round all day, feet up on the seats, chatting and smoking. Sometimes we went to Park Lane. Once we went to the Playboy Club and hung around until we were thrown out. Hyde Park Corner with its soapbox loonies was always good for a laugh.

The thing I liked best about school was the underpass I had to walk through in order to get there. Well, it wasn't really the underpass that I loved, it was the busker who was always there. He played Lou Reed, Leonard Cohen, Ralph McTell – music to slit your wrists by. His calling voice echoed in the underpass, and his songs wept. They prayed. He never knew it, but he healed my soul.

I discovered Zionism in London. At Habonim, a Jewish youth movement, I developed yet another secret life. I became a proud Jew who dreamed of living the life of a pioneer in the land of Israel. I watched and re-watched *Exodus* the movie, imagining myself as Karen, the teenage Holocaust survivor fighting for a new life in the Promised Land.

Strangely in these years, when I was comparatively fearless and prepared to expose myself to danger, the amount of uninvited traumas in my life dwindled. I smoked, drank, and drugged my way through my teens and my early twenties. During a brief stay in Australia, between England and America, when I was fourteen going on fifteen, I hung out with university students, dropped acid, marched in anti-Vietnam demonstrations, bought matchboxes filled with dope on the steps of Flinders Street Station, heard Allen Ginsburg read *Howl* at Melbourne Town Hall, and tried to avoid accompanying my mother, stepfather and Aviva to America by running away from home. I went from Melbourne all the way to Adelaide, but they found me and brought me back. A year later, in America, just before my sixteenth birthday, I lost my virginity. Yep, I was a wild one for a while, but despite all the craziness I tend to look back on those years as quiet. I did a lot, caused a lot, but other than being attacked by a watchdog at an archaeological dig in Caesarea a few years before I met Jack, nothing much happened to me.

I was at the tail end of my crazy years when I met Jack at a party in Jerusalem. We seemed to fit, but by the time we had our first child I was losing interest in drugs and parties and motorbikes. Jack is a difficult person, but a good one. He never deceived me. It was I who changed, not he.

9

Those two nights between the biopsies and the results I lay in bed and worried about all the sleep I'd lost. I worried about having used sweetener in my tea. I worried about all the coffee I'd drunk before I quit. I worried about having overworked. I worried about having eaten all that red meat when the doctor told me my iron was low. I worried about the weight I'd put on. I worried about all the cigarettes I'd smoked in my youth. I worried about the drugs I'd taken all those years ago. It was hard, impossible to believe, but I might have cancer. CANCER. The very word set my teeth on edge. I'd never been able to say the word in anything louder than a whisper. I'd never been able to think of it without feeling a weakness in my bones. How could this be happening to me?

Friday morning saw us back in the waiting room of the breast-screen clinic. There were five couples, including Doug and me, holding hands, staring blankly or flicking through magazines. One couple was not holding hands. The woman, older than I, was haranguing her husband. She looked incredibly tense, ready to snap. Apparently they'd parked in a no-standing zone, and now that they'd arrived and registered, he wanted to go back to move the car.

"That's right," she hissed. "Just piss off right when I need you."

"But the car," he whispered meekly.

"Bugger the car!"

The receptionist looked up.

"You're running away again, plain and simple." The hiss was now clearly audible. "Go on then. Piss off and leave me alone."

Her husband slunk out, hands shoved in the pockets of his jacket.

Doug and I held hands. I've always loved Doug's hands. I noticed them first when we were courting, when he sat at my kitchen table and read me a poem he'd written. I listened to the poem and looked at his hands, holding the paper. They were a poet's hands, strong, fine, dark. The fingers were long and slim, but there was nothing effeminate about those hands. They were beautiful. They were powerful. They were wise. I took comfort in them now, as the minutes slowly ticked by.

One couple was called in to see the doctor. They were young, and worried. They emerged less than ten minutes later, radiant, smiling, arms around each other, a bit like victors in a doubles tennis tournament. The door closed behind them with a slight bang, and all I could think was that their good fortune lowered my chances of success. As if the five couples in that waiting room on that autumnal Friday morning surely represented the breast cancer statistics of a nation.

The browbeaten husband returned just in time to be ushered into the doctor's office with his terrified wife. Doug and I sat silently with the other remaining couple, an elderly man and woman, both quite stately. This must be how a prisoner feels, I thought, while the jury deliberates. My fate was hanging in the balance, and there was absolutely nothing I could do. The anxiety was becoming physically painful. My breathing was labored.

Twenty minutes later, the couple emerged, escorted by a nurse. The woman was sobbing, her head was bowed. Her husband had his arm around her rather ample waist as the nurse let them into another room.

Our turn. My heart thumped. We were shown into the doctor's surgery. I was hoping it would be Elizabeth's mother, the woman who'd done the biopsies, but it was a man. He looked stern and overworked. A nurse came in after him and sat near me. My heart sank. The nurses were busy. They would only be attending women who needed further treatment. She wouldn't be here if the news was good.

The doctor pinned a scan up on the X-ray board.

"You have breast cancer," he said, matter-of-factly. No apology. No "I'm afraid." No hesitation. "You have breast cancer." Just like that. I slumped in my seat, shaking all over.

"No," I said. "No. No."

"Oh yes you do," he said, rather impatiently. I was just one of many he'd say this to today. "Look." He tapped the scan. "Left breast. Here," he tapped, "at five o'clock. Seven centimeters. And here." Tap. "At one o'clock. Five centimeters. And here." Tap. "Pre-cancerous growth at three o'clock."

"No," I said. "No." I didn't even know what he meant with all the clock references. The nurse didn't move.

"Look," says he. "I don't have time for this. You need to see a breast surgeon. Arrange a mastectomy. My work with you is done."

And that was my introduction to the world of breast cancer.

Doug and the nurse helped me from my chair, and out we went, through the waiting room, me sobbing on Doug's shoulder, the remaining couple frozen in terror.

"I need to give you some literature," said the nurse.

"Not here," I replied. "I need to get out of here."

Doug and I waited outside while she gathered the requisite government booklets on breast cancer. What to do next. Mastectomies, lumpectomies, breast reconstruction. Various options. How to tell the kids. Living with uncertainty. Blablablabla.

The nurse hovered. "Do you need help finding a breast surgeon?"

"Let's call Andrew," I said to Doug. "He'll recommend someone." For a moment, I unslumped. I was moving on, contemplating the next step. I wanted to put a lot of distance between us and the breast-screen clinic with its sterile waiting room and its long biopsy needles and its heartless doctor. I wanted to be somewhere else.

"Wait," said Doug. He turned to the nurse. "I want to see her file. I want you to make sure that you haven't confused her with another Deborah Miller. It's a common name."

The nurse obliged. She was a sweet woman. She disappeared into the clinic and emerged with a file. "See," she showed us. "Deborah Miller. Date of birth, September 27, 1957." My name, my date of birth, my address. My biopsy results. As the nurse left, I pulled out my mobile phone and called Andrew.

I'd never been a fan of mobile phones. Never really had much use for them, except to keep track of the kids. During the next few weeks, however, in the flurry of appointment-making, they would prove to be my lifeline. Oh, yes. There was that one other time. Yes, I remember. Last year, when I was in the bunker, in Safed. I wouldn't let go of my phone.

Andrew was wonderful. Within minutes he'd contacted a breast surgeon at the Worthington Hospital who would see us in a few hours.

"She's good," he said. "One of the best."

I think we were both in a state of shock, but Doug seemed to be holding it together. He steered me to the car and drove with one hand, holding mine with the other. I was still clasping my mobile phone, the way I had in the bunker in Safed. How could this be happening? How was I going to get through it? We were in a dark tunnel. I'd always feared absolute darkness. I'd always slept with a crack of light coming from somewhere.

We needed a referral from a GP to take to the breast surgeon. The GP who'd prescribed red meat for my iron deficiency was nearby. It was a quiet suburban practice in an old brick home, something timeless about it. It could have been a doctor's office from my childhood. Doug told the receptionist what had happened and we were squeezed in between patients.

The doctor, a woman on the verge of retirement, was shocked. I guess she was sympathetic, but I was not open to sympathy. I didn't want sympathy. I wanted someone to pull the plug, to tell me this wasn't happening, that it was all a big mistake. I wanted someone to pull me out from under the car.

As she wrote the referral I heard myself demanding a prescription for sleeping pills. I'd never demanded anything from a doctor. I'd never taken a sleeping pill in my life. I'd endured three decades of sleeplessness, but now I had cancer. CANCER. I needed pills. I needed to check out. The thought of lying awake all night with my thoughts was unbearable. Unbearable. How was this to be borne?

"I'm having trouble breathing," I said to the GP. "There's something wrong in my chest!"

"It's probably anxiety," she said. "But be sure to tell the breast surgeon."

Worthington Hospital was on the other side of town, so we decided to go straight there. I think we just wanted to keep moving. What was the point in going home first? I couldn't see a point in anything. Everything was a blur, pointless. My whole life was collapsing like a deck of cards. Fallen in disarray.

The Worthington is a tallish, greyish building in a busy commercial neighborhood. It took us twenty minutes to find a parking space. Or maybe it was five. What was time? I had cancer.

The breast surgeon was on the fifth floor. I know her name. I know the name of the GP as well. I could describe them for you, try to give you a sense of who they are, but I don't want to. It would be stressful, like trying to make out shapes in the dark. Their only role in this story is as "the GP" and "the breast surgeon."

The breast surgeon's rooms were very modern, with Rothko reproductions on the walls. As we waited in the reception with the oversized envelope containing my breast scans, a young woman emerged from the consulting room, holding hers.

"It's so sudden," she said to the receptionist. "I've got four children, and there's my job…I don't know how I'm going to juggle this." Her voice was shrill. She seemed so young, and quite petite. How could she bear it?

We were invited in. The breast surgeon looked at my scans, and took control. Thank God. At last.

"It looks quite simple," she said. "The two lesions are too far apart for a lumpectomy. It'll have to be a mastectomy. That means I'll have to remove the whole breast."

Take it, I thought, and good riddance. The breast that suckled my children had betrayed me. It was trying to kill me. I didn't want it any more.

"This appears to be a simple case of early breast cancer," she continued. "When I remove the breast I'll check the glands. My guess is that it hasn't progressed to the glands, but if it has, we'll remove them too. Simple. A mastectomy is not a complex operation. You'll need about three weeks' recovery time."

"That's it?" I asked.

"Well," she said, "you could have some chemotherapy, but I doubt that will be necessary. I'd probably recommend a course of radiotherapy, which would kill off any stray cancer cells that may have been missed in the operation. It's just precautionary, but I'd recommend it for peace of mind."

Chemotherapy. Radiation. I knew the words, but apart from bald heads and annual telethons, I had no idea what they meant. I'd never read about people having chemo, never seen pictures. I had no idea what it entailed. I'd always steered well clear of that sort of thing. It was depressing. And scary.

"Radiation's painless," she said. "Most people just feel a bit lethargic afterwards. Odds are, that'll be the end of it. The vast majority of women never have a recurrence."

Really? That was it? I wasn't going to die next week, or next month, or next year? Losing a breast seemed quite tolerable under the circumstances. I was eager to get on with it. I tried to take a deep breath, and felt my chest rattle.

"But my chest," I said. "There's something wrong. I'm rasping when I breathe."

"Okay. We'll do an X-ray and CT scan tomorrow, but I'd say it's not related to the breast cancer. Breathlessness is a sign of late-stage cancer, and these scans clearly indicate that we've caught yours early."

We discussed the possibility of breast reconstruction directly after the mastectomy. I said no, I'd rather wait and decide at a later date, so Doug and I were ushered into another room to discuss prosthetic breasts and mastectomy bras with a breast care nurse. I hadn't had so much attention paid to my breasts since my babies had clutched them between their tiny hands and sucked noisily at the nipples.

The X-ray and CT scan were booked for the following day, and off we went, home in the rush-hour traffic.

I didn't look at the impatient travelers in the other cars. I didn't look at the grey Melbourne streets. I looked at the sky, inky with evening, and at the branches of the autumn trees so well defined against it. This was life. Why had I never seen it in this way? Why had I never realized that it could just disappear, that it could end, just like that? I'd been afraid many times, but I'd never really understood the fragility of life.

Once, during one of those childhood summers in Singapore, I saved a man's life. I was swimming at the Tanglin Club with my mother and stepfather. In those days there were very few Anglos in Singapore, and membership at the Tanglin Club was a must for anyone with any sense of high society. I'd made a friend in the water, as nine-year-old girls tend to do, and we were diving for coins. One of us would throw a coin into the pool and when it settled on the bottom, the other would try to retrieve it. My friend threw the coin and before I dived for it I noticed someone lying on the bottom of the pool. I didn't pay much attention. I thought it was a boy playing dead. They often did that, while their friends timed them to see how long they could last before coming up for air. The coin fell near the prone figure, and as I dived beneath the surface and neared the bottom of the pool I saw that it wasn't a boy. It was a man, an older man, but not just his hair was grey. He was grey all over, bluish grey, and unconscious. His lips were swollen. I shot back to the surface and screamed, pointing to the figure way down there at the bottom of the deep end. Within seconds a young man had dived in and was carrying him to the surface. They laid him on the fake grass and resuscitated him before the ambulance arrived. He survived. There was a news item about the incident in the *Straits Times* the following day. The man who pulled him out of the pool was the real hero, but I rated a mention.

I will never forget the drowning man's blue-grey face as he lay near death at the bottom of the pool at the Tanglin Club, in downtown Singapore, on that bright December day. He was lost in breathless silence while, above, music blared, children laughed, and Anglo parents browned themselves on deckchairs, sipping fancy drinks with paper umbrellas in them. Above, it was a near-perfect day in the tropics, blue skies and gentle breeze, the air fragrant with last night's rain, but the bottom of the pool was cold, silent, dead.

10

I called my mother and asked her to meet us at home. My mother is a busy woman. When she acquiesced without question, I realized that she must already know. The story about the strained shoulder hadn't fooled her. I was also a mother. I understood. Poor mum. This would really pull the rug out from under her.

Since my stepfather had died ten years earlier, my mother had worked hard at filling up her life, at staying very busy. And she'd done a magnificent job. I was proud of her. Instead of indulging in the blues of widowhood, she had bounced back and made a life for herself. In many ways, as she noted in her seventieth-birthday speech, these years of widowhood had been the richest of her life. She'd been a wife since she was nineteen and still at home. This was her very first taste of real independence.

My stepfather, an Englishman with Richard Burton's voice and looks and a towering intellect, had kind of stolen the show during their marriage. He was the sort of man to whom one paid attention. People were drawn to him. He understood the new physics. He bought and mastered one of the first computers on the market. He was a master chess player, a phenomenal bridge partner. He could recite reams of poetry from memory. Keats, Shakespeare, Eliot, Pound. The whole of *The Rime of the Ancient Mariner*, all in that wonderfully theatrical English accent. He was a true Renaissance man. When I was a teenager, a few of my girlfriends fell in love with him. I think he enjoyed that. He suffered his final illness not only stoically, but joyfully, determined to savor every moment of this ultimate human experience.

The cancer first appeared as a melanoma in his eye. The eye was removed and replaced with glass. Then it spread to the brain. Chemo failed, and he was given three or four months. He took them with glee. He resumed smoking his luxury Dunhills and splurged on expensive chocolates and Veuve Clicquot champagne. He staged his own wake, inviting family and friends to listen to his reflections on life. Even in his waning, people were attracted to him. They came and they came again, unnaturally drawn to a home in which death was in progress. He was like a magnet, outrageous, entertaining, profound. My mother, for all her dark good looks and fiery personality, lived in his shadow. When he died she was lost, disincorporated; but slowly, slowly she picked up the pieces, put herself back together, tested her wings, and flew. It took time, a couple of years. She was unpartnered for the first time in fifty years, and as long as she was busy to the point of distraction, it worked.

She was there when we arrived, sitting at the kitchen table. She took one look at my face and let out a sob. Her face crumpled and she looked her age.

"What is it?" she asked, redundantly.

"Breast cancer, but it's early. I'm having a mastectomy and odds are everything will be fine."

My mother got that serious, problem-solving look on her face. Who had I seen? Will I get a second opinion? Her questions irritated me. They seemed so utterly beside the point.

We needed to tell the children. I had no idea how. One of the booklets I'd been given had a chapter on it. Young children. Older children. Adult children. My youngest, Ben, had just turned fifteen. My daughter, Orly, would be eighteen in another month. My oldest, David, was twenty. I guess they came in the "older children" category. "Be honest," I read. "Don't leave them guessing, but you can also be positive. Point out to them that early breast cancer has a very high survival rate."

My three children are same same but different. They are obviously siblings. Their faces share a certain way of looking out at the world. But David is tall, with an even taller intellect and a mix of streetwise cynicism and openhearted naivety that never fails to astound me. Everyone says he will go far. He's already come a very long way. Orly is petite, fiery, brilliant, beautiful. A girl-becoming-woman with skin so soft, it begs to be stroked. She is quick-minded and quick-tempered, my darling daughter. And Benny, who will always be my baby, is a broad-shouldered, handsome, dimply, smiley kid who loves his footy and his cricket and loves whom he loves with a heart of liquid gold.

What would I have said about my three kids back then, two and a half years ago, when I was preparing to tell them that I had breast cancer? Not the above. My family was troubled. Rabbi Hoffman says that all families are troubled, some just hide it better than others. He says the ones who hide it best, the ones who present a shiny face to the world, the teacher's-pet families, are often the most troubled, covering up the darkest secrets. Tolstoy said that troubled families were at least interesting. I took some comfort in that. Each of my kids had problems. I had problems. My mother had problems. Doug had problems. We were problematic.

When Doug entered my life, a few years before my diagnosis, we were a dysfunctional family. I'd been soldiering on as a single parent for years. I managed to maintain the veneer by cooking their meals, making their school lunches, making their beds, washing their clothes (I never ironed), doing their dishes, taking out their rubbish, and keeping myself, my inner life, well away, as if it were a jewel too precious for them to touch. They might soil it or scratch it or break it. I was a mother on automatic pilot. I shopped for them, I drove them to school, to their friends' houses. I picked them up and took them to their swimming lessons and their ballet classes and their karate, always in a hurry, always hurrying them. I rarely played with them. I didn't sit with them in the evenings and watch TV or guide them through their homework. Who had the time? Who had the emotional energy? In a way, in the things that counted, we lived separate lives.

Within two years of my divorce they were eating dinner in front of the TV every night, except Fridays. Sabbath eve. I held onto Friday nights, thank God. On Friday nights I made roast chicken and invited guests and we'd sit together in the dining room, like a real family. Am I being too harsh? Probably. We had our share of good times. But we did have serious problems. Benny was sad and obstreperous. Orly was angry. David was veering out of control, and I was remote. I was on remote control. Inside, I was swimming in the deep blue seas of Torah. I was doing my best to lose myself, to hide myself in desert springs and fields of holy apples.

When Doug entered our lives he would not, he could not, allow things to remain the way they were. He wanted clear boundaries, and he was right. We had none. I guess I'd been a good enough mother, barring the bouts of emotional unavailability, but

I was a lousy father. Doug wanted rules. He wanted consequences. It was an uphill battle. A number of times, he threw up his hands in despair – no, in sullen, silent fury – and gave up. He wouldn't communicate with one or other of the kids for weeks. Once he moved out altogether. We met on weekends at the park, as he refused to set foot in the house. And who could blame him? The kids were often outrageous. They could be brats, especially when they felt encroached upon. They weren't used to boundaries.

Doug, who is a good man, always came back, and tried again, and slowly, slowly, imperceptibly, the kids' resentment of this intruder, this usurper who was trying to change everything, began to soften and transform. At times I thought that his standards were too high, that he wanted an unattainable ideal. Perhaps we've both also softened over the years. I've come to appreciate that what he wanted, what he wants, is something to aim for, and the closer we get, the closer we come to being a family. It's been hard for him. The two years we'd been together prior to the diagnosis had already felt like multiple lifetimes. Each of the kids had had their crises, one of them major. And they'd witnessed their father's drug-fueled nervous breakdown, in our living room, at a Passover meal for the extended family, the day before Doug and I had our first real get-to-know-you conversation.

But that's another story. There are too many stories, too many rivers and rivulets and creeks. This story is about my cancer, it's about the ocean where all the rivers meet, and at this point in the story I was struggling for breath, coughing and rattling while my mother worried and Doug, God bless him, called the kids into the kitchen.

They saw our serious faces, and were quiet. I explained the situation matter-of-factly, as if it was a matter of fact. Doug filled in a few details. I'd be in hospital for a while, then at home resting. Everyone would have to pitch in and help. We left the question of death hanging, unasked, in limbo. And so my family began a new phase of its life.

When I finally collapsed into bed that night, exhausted, I could barely breathe. Doug propped me up on pillows, I took my first ever sleeping pill and I slept half-sitting, fitfully. The night was full of demons, shadowy fears. If I dreamed I didn't know it.

The following day we returned to the Worthington, to the search for a parking spot, and on to the Department of Nuclear Medicine. Nuclear medicine. What were they going to do to me? The waiting room was crowded. A popular soap opera blared from a TV attached to the wall. Young doctor with strong chiseled jawline bends over beautiful young female patient, while pretty nurse, obviously in love with doctor, hovers within reach. Beautiful young patient is deathly pale. Her ashen lips are slightly parted. Her eyelids flicker. "There's not much more we can do," says handsome doctor in low sexy voice. His brow is furrowed with concern. "It's up to her now." Nurse sneaks a squeeze of doctor's broad manly shoulder and the music swells…

It was all too ridiculous. Couldn't they at least change the station? Surely there was some news to report, a natural disaster, a terrorist attack, a famine. The farcical hospital drama was being watched by a roomful of people waiting to be scanned for cancer, or TB or God knows what. For all my desire to be young and pretty, I didn't want a ghost-white face and ashen lips. Doug and I stole a smile at the absurdity of it. He squeezed my hand.

My turn. I was led down a corridor to a room dominated by a giant tubular machine. So this was a CT. I'd seen them on TV. I didn't even try to chat. I was tired, very tired. I undressed behind the curtain and put on their ridiculous hospital gown, green of course. The young technician, not nearly as handsome as the TV doctor, was flirting with his pretty enough assistant. I lay back on the bed that fed into the tube with relief. I was so tired. The pair left the room and the tube moved toward me, or my bed moved toward the tube. I've had many scans since then, and I still don't remember.

A disembodied voice commanded, "Take a deep breath and hold!" Hold, hold. I tried counting down in my head. My lungs were bursting. I couldn't do it.

"Breathe freely!" Thank God. Thank God.

"Take a deep breath and hold!" Oh dear God, again? I couldn't, I couldn't.

"Breathe freely." I gasped and gulped in air, oxygen, life, grateful as a Bedouin at an oasis.

The pair returned. "How are your veins? I need to inject some dye."

I stared mutely. "The major problem with cancer patients," he said to his nearly pretty assistant, "is tired veins."

I meekly held out my arm. So this was my future. Cancer patient with tired veins.

"Idiot!" I wanted to scream. "I've never done this before. I'm scared of needles. Can't you see? I'm *not* a *cancer patient*!"

Instead I stared mutely. The needle slipped in. The dye was cast. I tasted metal and felt as if I'd peed my pants. The duo exited again, rather gaily, and I was left to a repeat of the breath-holding torture, and finally it was over. I was gasping so much I could hardly re-dress.

After the CT scan, the X-ray passed in a haze. I took Doug's arm and begged him to take me home. It took us over an hour in rush-hour traffic.

Another restless, dreamless night, dozing, half-sitting, my lungs pleading for air. What was going on? I felt as if I was sinking, drowning.

Doug and I returned to the breast surgeon the following afternoon. A few minutes after her previous patient had left she emerged from her office and, instead of asking us in, dashed past us. She didn't return for forty minutes. We sat, silent, holding hands, worrying. Finally, we gathered in her office.

"I can't do the mastectomy," she said. "We've found some problems with your lungs."

Dread washed over me. My mouth fell open.

"A number of suspicious areas appear on the scans. You have fluid on both lungs. It could be an infection, or it could be cancer. Either way, you're very sick. I've referred you to a respiratory specialist. He's good, one of the best. He'll see you tomorrow, due to the urgency."

I cracked. I crumpled. "No! No!" I cried. I bawled.

And something strange happened.

She got angry. The fancy breast surgeon in her Worthington Hospital suite with the million-dollar view yelled at me. "Stop crying! There's nothing I can do! I've been sitting downstairs with the radiologist who did your scans for the best part of an hour. It's all there."

The doctor who'd given me the initial diagnosis had also been angry. "See?" he'd cried, tapping the scans. "Here, and here. There's nothing I can do. You need a breast surgeon."

Why were they angry? Is that how they protect themselves from all this misery? In the movies, in the novels, bad news like this was delivered with tact. The music swells, and the weeping, stricken heroine is comforted.

This woman, who had just told me I had fluid on my lungs, and other things I didn't understand and didn't want to know about, was shouting at me.

The health care nurse, the one who the previous day had advised us on government rebates for a prosthetic breast, ushered us out of the room and gave us the details for my appointment with the respiratory doctor. She seemed unsettled by the breast surgeon's outburst.

I never wanted to see the breast surgeon again, and I didn't. I moved on, and shoved the incident away in the larger part of my mind labeled "things to be dealt with later." Months later, just before Christmas, I received a card from her. She hoped I was doing well and sent good wishes. It wasn't an apology, but I guess it was the best she could do.

I was gasping and rattling when we left the breast surgeon's suite. Doug left me sitting in the hospital foyer and brought the car to the entrance. On the way home we tried to discuss the situation. The lung issues were obviously serious, but they were probably unrelated. I must have picked up an infection. It would all work out. We needed to have faith. I looked at the sky, at the darkish clouds. Perhaps it would rain. The leaves on the trees were exquisite, each one a masterpiece. A small flock of seagulls flew by, heading for the ocean. Suddenly, I wanted to be near the sea, to look out over the ocean, to spread my wings over it all, to own it, to keep it. It was all too precious. I was crying again.

"Put my tears in Your bottle: they are already in Your book." I whispered this line from Psalms that night, when Doug was sleeping beside me. I was half-sitting again, propped up by pillows, wheezing and crying. Now that I'd been told there was something seriously wrong with my lungs I allowed myself to feel the full force of whatever it was. It was time to stop pretending. I was out of energy, out of breath, and I was seriously ill. It was a relief to know I didn't have to keep going any more. I could rest. At least that.

Again I swam in and out of sleep, going under, wanting to let go, to wander free deep beneath the surface, but I re-emerged, with a gasp. Bathed in sweat. Listening to the night sounds. A solitary passing car. A possum running across the roof. A silence full of questions. And I went under again, to that place where the silence is solid and whispers are not heard.

I'd been having night sweats for weeks, waking up soaked through and needing to change my pajamas. Before my diagnosis I'd been told it was menopause. Now I was being told it was probably due to infection. It couldn't be cancer. Night sweats like that are a sign of a very late stage, and I wasn't late stage.

Next morning we drove to Dr. Landsdowne, the respiratory specialist. He was in another part of town, in a leafy wealthy suburb. The bulk of his patients seemed to be asthmatics, mostly children. He listened to my chest and looked at the scans. I told him, breathlessly, that I couldn't stop gasping.

"It could be an infection," he said. "Possibly TB."

He sent me for a blood test and called me at home a few hours later. The blood test was inconclusive. Some fluid would have to be extracted from my lung.

We were back at the Worthington that afternoon. So much for resting. Well, I did rest in a manner of speaking. I sat slumped over a kind of cushioned barrel while fluid was extracted from my lung by a syringe inserted through my back. It sounds awful, but I don't remember it hurting. The doctor showed me a flask nearly full of pinkish fluid.

"So much!" I gasped.

"This is just a sample. There's a lot more where that came from."

Oy. But he was a nice man, gently funny, and kind. And I don't remember it hurting.

We went home to await the results. I might have picked up TB years earlier. I might have been carrying it for decades. It might have manifested now, when my resistance was lowered by the breast cancer. It was possible. If it was TB, I'd go on a lengthy course of antibiotics. Then I'd have the mastectomy and that would be that. I lay in bed, staring at a crack of light. Please God, let me have TB. Please let me have TB. Please, please, not cancer in my lungs.

The respiratory doctor called the following afternoon. The tests on the fluid were inconclusive. It seemed to be an infection, it had some characteristics of an infection, but they couldn't be sure. I needed to have a bronchoscopy, the following morning, at the Worthington.

If he shoved a bronchoscope down my throat and into my airways, he could have a look at my lungs, and extract more fluid. Great.

11

Doug and I were buried in our world of tests, of waiting and praying. Outside, in the world we once inhabited, all hell was breaking loose. The news was spreading. Emails flooded my inbox. The letter box filled with cards. Food and flowers were left at the door. A few brave souls telephoned. I couldn't deal with it. I was drowning.

I'd canceled my scheduled classes and lectures. Our life now was all about keeping up with the tide of tests, struggling to ride the wave, but knowing deep down that we were about to be dumped.

The bronchoscopy involved a light general anesthetic. I signed in as a day patient, and we waited in a huge lobby with a crowd of others to be called by the anesthetist for a consultation. I think we waited for more than an hour. I'd stopped bringing my own books to read and I refused to stoop to magazines or the wall TV, so I stared at my hands, looked at the pictures on the walls. Mostly, I surreptitiously studied the people around me. For the first time in years I had the opportunity, the luxury to look around. I'd been so caught up in my own little world, my tiny, endless universe of Torah, worlds within worlds. Even when I did get away from the books and the computer screen, usually to the supermarket, I'd barely noticed the people around me. I'd forgotten how interesting they could be. Now I strained to hear their huddled conversations, I studied their looks, and I imagined their lives. I guess it helped me to forget my own.

My name was called and we rose, but the anesthetist showed Doug the palm of her hand.

"I'll see her alone," she said imperiously. Doug went back to his seat and I meekly followed her into a cubicle of a consulting room.

When we were seated she took out a clipboard and asked me what by now were becoming routine questions about my health. I was shocked to see her hands. The fingers were gnarled and bent. Arthritis? It looked painful. How would those fingers find my vein? How could they possibly be gentle, agile, precise? She could barely wield a pen! She pulled out a stethoscope and listened to my back.

"I don't detect anything," she remarked.

"Surely that's a good sign?" I asked hopefully. "Do you think it could be an infection?"

"Does it matter?" she asked.

I was doubly shocked. "Of course it matters. I don't want to have secondary cancer. That's a death sentence. I couldn't bear it. I couldn't bear it." My eyes leaked a few tears. They had been readily available for days, and every so often they dropped out when I didn't have the strength to keep the tap screwed tight.

The anesthetist was a majestic woman – perhaps some sort of elder. She was gnarled and old, and possibly wise.

She slammed her crooked hands down on the desk, startling me.

"Oh yes you could! Oh yes you will!"

I froze, like I had when I'd been hauled in front of Miss Mountain, my primary school headmistress, a severe woman who was worshiped as a god by staff and students. Her displeasure was the mark of Cain.

"What are you afraid of?" the anesthetist demanded.

"I'm afraid of having cancer," I replied tearily. I wished she'd take me in her old wise arms and make it all go away.

"No!" her voice was an urgent hiss. She caught my eyes and held them. Her eyes were narrow, and passionate. And loving. I was frightened.

"You're afraid of the future. You're afraid of tomorrow. You're afraid of this afternoon. What is that? Nothing! All any of us have is right now. What are you afraid of right now?"

I wanted to say I was afraid of the cancer, of what would happen to me, but that wasn't right now, so I shut up. My fear was turning to anger. How dare she accost me like this, as if she had all the answers? She had no right, no right. I gathered my things and walked out, wheezing and gasping, with a feeble attempt at holding my head high. I was shaken.

Doug and I were shown into pre-op, into a recliner chair surrounded by curtains. I'd tried to tell Doug about the anesthetist, but it came out all jumbled. Dr. Landsdowne showed up and said something encouraging before going to scrub up.

A nurse gave me an injection, some kind of relaxant, and within seconds I was high. And within seconds I finally understood. The anesthetist was right. She was a wise, wise woman, a mystic. She knew the secrets of this dark place, this abyss into which I'd been tossed. She knew where the light was. There is only now. Fear is a fiction. I was led into the operating room by the nurse. Dr. Landsdowne and the anesthetist were waiting, beckoning me to the waiting operating table. But I disentangled myself from the nurse and headed for the wise woman, the elder disguised as an anesthetist.

"You're right!" I was awestruck, radiant. "There is only now!" I stepped closer and hugged her.

I smiled. I beamed. The dark clouds had drifted away. The clarity was brilliant. The gnarled hands that guided the needle into my wrist were sure and steady and gentle. And wise. I never felt the drip go in.

I awoke in post-op, coughing. I was underwater again, way down. Everything was swimming around me, above me. I was sinking. The anesthetist said something to me. I suppose I responded, because she turned and walked away. I couldn't clear my head. I felt like a dog trying to shake itself out of a nightmare. I wanted Doug.

"Not yet, darling," said the nurse. "We'll wait a bit longer, till you're more alert."

My throat ached. I tried to prop myself up on my elbows, but fell back on the bed, exhausted. As my head cleared, I remembered the anesthetist's words. All the joy was gone. It was just some more new-age crap. Of course I was afraid. Who wouldn't be?

I know the answer to that.

"Yea, though I walk through the valley of the shadow of death, I will fear no evil, for You are with me, Your rod and Your staff they comfort me…"

The Rebbe of Piacezna was not afraid. He'd lost his entire family, his nation was in ruins, yet in the heart of the fury he wrote the most sublime Torah. He wrote of revelation and sanctification in the stinking pit of the twentieth century. His words were like sweetest incense rising up to heaven from a pile of ashes. But the Rebbe was a holy man. He was exceptional. How could someone like me not be afraid?

I remembered a book Rabbi Hoffman had recommended a few years back. It was written by a man who called himself "Ka Tzetnik," which simply means "concentration camp inmate," followed by his number, "1345633." He said this was not a pen name. It was what his time in Auschwitz had made him. This man had been plagued by nightmares for years, for decades, night after night, since the war. In desperation he traveled to Holland to try "psychedelic psychotherapy." Under the influence of LSD he revisited Auschwitz in his mind, only this time the Hebrew word *Shiviti*, from the psalm that begins "I have set the Lord always before me," hovered above him in air thick with the ashes of human flesh. The *Shiviti*, crafted as a decorative plaque, is usually hung in a synagogue to encourage contemplative prayer. Years after the fact, Yehiel DeNur, aka Ka Tzetnik, achieved some sort of revelation with the help of LSD, but back then, in the living hell, surely he was afraid.

What were my troubles against these? True, I was very ill, but I had all the advantages of modern medicine, all the comforts of a caring community. And anyway, it might not be that bad. Perhaps I only had TB. Perhaps the cancer was still in its early stages. Please God, let it be TB.

Doug and I returned home, to the waiting game. Dr. Landsdowne had promised to call with the results the following afternoon. The day was weary with worry. I jumped whenever the phone rang.

He called late in the afternoon.

"The results of the bronchoscopy are inconclusive. I'm afraid you need a lung biopsy. I've booked you in at the Worthington. I've got you a good surgeon, one of the best. You'll be in hospital for at least three days while we drain the fluid from your lungs. It's not a pleasant operation, but the results will be conclusive."

Doug was up in arms. This was a serious operation. I could be feeling the effects for months, maybe years. He took me to a Chinese doctor. She asked me questions, looked at my eyes and my tongue.

"It's an infection," she said. "I'm sure of it. There's no cancer in your lungs. But your kidneys aren't the best. I can give you some herbs for that."

All the same, I wanted the biopsy. I insisted. Doug was not happy, but he took me back to the Worthington, to meet the surgeon and schedule the operation. As I struggled to keep pace with the surgeon as he led us to his office, he said, "A woman your age shouldn't be struggling for breath like that." I took it as a criticism. The operation was scheduled for the following day. They weren't wasting any time. I had to conclude that I may not have much time.

We drove home through the neighborhood in which I'd spent my formative years, right past the spot where I'd been run over, and along the banks of the Yarra, the comfortingly familiar river that winds through the heart of Melbourne. These were the scenes of my childhood: the park, the tennis courts, the brown snaky water, the bridges, the city skyline. The neon skipping girl high on a billboard advertising vinegar. Not much had changed. I had changed. I had cancer. How many more times would I see this river, these trees, this bridge? We stopped at the lights and I watched the joggers on the riverbank. I could barely walk from the car to the curb. I could barely breathe. I envied them their agility, their strength, their health, their breath.

The day before I'd called a childhood friend, now an oncologist who specialized in palliative care. I told him I couldn't breathe, begged him to help. I'd been given codeine, and an inhaler for asthmatics. Nothing worked. I didn't have enough breath, and what I had I couldn't catch.

"That's ridiculous," he'd said. "It can't be. That's a major symptom of final-stage disease. It must be something else."

I was willing to go with the "something else," but meanwhile, I couldn't breathe.

"What can I do?" I asked. "I need breath."

"Well, liquid morphine would help, but surely it can't be that severe."

We'd called the GP, insisted she come to the house. I had no energy to drag myself anywhere, except to tests, and more tests.

The morphine helped, but even so, I was still gasping. The Hebrew word for breath is also the word for soul. Was my soul struggling to leave my body? Was I dying? I was taking the liquid morphine, which helped my lungs a little, but I wasn't happy. I wasn't stoned. I was still gasping, and I was weighed down with worry.

The joggers seemed so carefree. They were probably thinking about the rest of their day, about work, or children, or shopping. They might have thought they had serious problems. They might have money issues or they might be in the midst of a divorce. Or they might be having a stressful time at work or with the kids. So they jogged, they got the endorphins going. Watching them, I had to face how sick I was. I could barely walk. I signed in at the Worthington and we were shown to the ward. I could tell that Doug was apprehensive, that he was making an effort to remain calm and reassuring. He was allowed to accompany me into pre-op, where I was given some sort of sedative. The patients were lying there in rows, bodies waiting to be operated upon.

When I was wheeled to the entrance of the operating room, the anesthetist, a middle-aged man, examined my wrist, plunged in the needle, and asked me pleasantly if I had any children.

"Ye…" That was it. I was out. I don't remember waking up. There'd been too many tests, too much anesthetic. I remember Doug accompanying me as I was wheeled back to the ward. A chest tube was reinflating my lung and draining the fluid, but I wasn't aware of it, not yet. I dipped in and out of sleep. I felt nothing except, towards morning, a pressure on my bladder. The nurse brought me a bed pan.

In the morning I met my three roommates, all elderly women who had been in the ward for some time with a variety of respiratory problems. They were sweet and encouraging. They'd already lightened my mood when the surgeon appeared, smiling. He'd taken the biopsy, and we wouldn't have the results for a few days, but everything he saw while operating indicated an infection. Yes, he felt sure that it was an infection, that the breast cancer was early stage.

Whoopee! My body was no longer numb. It was feeling good. It was brimming, overflowing with joy, with gratitude, with relief. Thank you God, oh thank you. God is good! God is great! I'm going to live! After the surgeon left, my roommates celebrated with me, such caring, kindly women, sitting on chairs next to their beds, reading, knitting, chatting, now and then taking oxygen from a mask.

It was Saturday morning, Shabbat, the holy Sabbath, and I felt reborn. I sneaked a call to Doug, who doesn't travel on Shabbat, and the news spread fast, reaching my congregation before the end of the morning service. During the week, they had held a special prayer service for me. They wanted to storm the gates of heaven, to rail and beg on my behalf. Of course I wasn't there, I was barely aware that it was happening, but now I can picture them, singing, weeping, swaying, my beloved spiritual family, my friends, my fellow lovers of Torah.

That Sabbath, when they heard of my reprieve, they sang, they drummed on the lectern, they wept with joy. Of course I wasn't there, but I know they did, because I know them. We had discovered our love of Torah together, in the days of the dastardly rabbi. Most of them are younger than I, but in a sense we grew up together, we were forged in fire and we emerged, scathed but transformed.

I was still somewhat wasted on morphine, and I was elated. My roommates told me that the other half of the ward was for women recovering from mastectomies. That would be me, in just a few months! I'd lose a breast, and the cancer would be gone. I was the happiest woman alive.

The following day I was moved to a private room. I promised to visit my new friends as soon as I was ambulatory. As I came down from the morphine high, I became aware of the tube and the pain. I still had morphine on demand, from a self-serve pump attached to my drip, but I was not comfortable. I didn't care. I'd been reprieved! I had no idea how strange I looked with the tube coming out of my chest, draining fluid into a clear box on the floor. My poor children were very subdued when they saw me.

"Don't worry, kids," I assured them. "The results are great. You have no idea how bad it could have been. We're very lucky."

They could see that I was speaking from the heart, and they looked relieved.

Doug waited by my bed every night until I fell asleep, and he was already back by my side in the morning when I awoke. I have never had a partner like him. I felt pampered, and deeply loved. My ex-husband Jack, a good man, was simply incapable of that kind of care. His parents were both Holocaust survivors. His father had a wife and two little girls before the war. All killed. His mother was engaged, and bereaved. They met after the war and after a few years in the newly established Jewish state, they immigrated to Australia. They were both deeply damaged. She took barbiturates, and he took to bouts of anger. He worked in a shoe factory. Jack was their only child, and he was weighed down by their grief. At times I see that same pain in the eyes of our children. Apart from them, Jack does not have a living relative, anywhere. Hitler, may his name be obliterated, has a lot to answer for.

I was taken off the morphine pump. Every morning I was visited by a woman who gave me breathing exercises to assist my reinflating lung. I imagined trying to blow up a balloon. I'd never been very good at that. I was afraid it would pop. I preferred letting go and watching it whizz around the room and fall scrawny and deflated onto the floor.

I was permitted to get out of bed and walk to the bathroom and back. The nurse temporarily disengaged my tube and reattached it when I returned to bed. The whole procedure took about twenty minutes, just to relieve my bladder! And only my bladder. Constipation, hospitals and I were old friends.

On the third day, Doug and I took a walk around the ward. I visited my former roommates, still sitting, still knitting. I shuffled to the other side of the ward, where women were recovering from mastectomies. They had a beautiful view, much better than the respiratory patients.

"I'll be back," I told a passing nurse. "In just a few months. On *this* side!"

By the time we got back to my room I was in agony. I took some codeine and waited for relief. I didn't know then that pain from this biopsy would plague me for years.

12

On the fifth day I was pronounced well enough to go home. But first the tube had to be removed. I lay on my side with my eyes closed and the nurse started to pull, and pull. And pull. It felt as if a huge snake was being pulled out of me. It just went on and on. I opened one eye and saw Doug trying to remain calm. It must have looked awful, macabre, but it didn't hurt, not then. I had no way of knowing how much it would hurt later on.

Having the tube pulled out was a surreal experience. I've never enjoyed science fiction or horror movies. I've always steered clear of them, as I have of roller coasters, yet here I was, starring in my very own gruesome production. When the tube was out, a doctor closed the wound with a few stitches.

We waited a couple more hours. An X-ray confirmed that my lung had fully reinflated, and I was free to go. I was still in pain, and very weak, but I didn't care. The results were good, and that was all that mattered. The surgeon had said I probably had pleurisy. I'd take some antibiotics, I'd have the mastectomy. All would be well.

At home, I crawled into bed. It was good to be back. I was going to be fine. The kids were home, and my mother. They tucked me into bed, we talked, we laughed, and they left me to rest. I was lying happily propped by pillows when the phone rang. I answered it cheerily.

"Deborah, this is Dr. Landsdowne."

"Yes, yes, hello!"

"I have the biopsy results."

My skin crawled.

"I'm sorry, Deborah. The biopsy has confirmed metastatic cancer."

I shrieked. Doug came running.

"But he said…" I sobbed. "He told me…"

I collapsed into the pillows. Doug took the phone. He got a pen and paper and wrote down some details. I wept. I heard my mother cry out, one great cry of pain, of fear, from the kitchen. The kids came running. We were all on my bed, holding onto each other like shipwrecked travelers on a raft. I tried to get a grip, but what was there to say? Just a few days ago I'd told them, "You don't know how lucky we are. You have no idea how bad it could have been."

This was how bad it could have been. Metastatic breast cancer. A death sentence.

We were stuck in the overplayed mother-has-cancer scene at the end of the movie. "We'll be okay," I said shakily. "We'll get through. I'll get better."

Doug insisted it was a mistake, that the biopsy results were wrong.

Dr. Landsdowne had made an appointment for me with an oncologist, very good man, one of the best, at the Worthington. I was learning that they are always "one of the best."

Doug had had enough of doctors and he'd had enough of the Worthington Hospital. For the first time since this whole saga had begun, he refused to accompany me. He felt I'd taken the wrong path since deciding to have the biopsy and he couldn't support me. Every professional we'd consulted and every one of our medically trained friends had insisted that the biopsy was necessary, and that the results would be definitive. I felt angry with Doug for disagreeing. I've since learned to value his stubbornness.

In the Book of Genesis, when God proclaims "It is not good for man to be alone," He decides to make for him "a helper against him." That's a literal translation. The partner is not to be a yes-person, or even someone to complement him. No. The partner is someone who stands opposite, to find the vital creativity that is born of dialectic tension.

Doug is a helper against me. I overlook my children's shortcomings; he pinpoints them. I shove rubbish out of sight, into cupboards; he sorts and discards it. I put my faith in medical science; he reads the signs, looks for omens, but in accordance with his tradition never bases decisions upon them. Over the years, we have adapted. I've learned to make boundaries with the kids; he's learned to accept them as they are. He still tidies and discards, and I still overfill drawers and closets; but I look for omens, I try to read the signs, and he has faith in medical science. Because we love each other.

I returned to the Worthington with my friend Amira and my mother. Amira brought a notebook and pen, ready to take notes during our meeting with the oncologist. My mother brought a worried look. I brought nothing. I felt numb.

And now my pen hovers over the page. I'd rather leave it blank, white, full of possibility. I don't want to tell this part of the story. Perhaps I don't know how. How can I describe waiting for the oncologist, feeling numb, filling out forms, more forms, on the top floor of the Worthington, eight stories above a ground that I could not feel? The doctor's suite was plush, immaculate, nondescript, and sterile. The receptionist was expressionless. Upmarket magazines were piled neatly on the glass coffee table. The waiting room was silent, colorless, despite the Rothko prints on the walls. I was sick of the Worthington, and I was sick of Rothko prints. Doug thought they were a bad omen. Amira, my mother, and I sat quietly, grim-faced.

The oncologist was as nondescript as his consulting rooms. I don't remember his name. All I remember is that when he told us that I had metastatic disease, which was incurable, terminal, but in certain cases could be controlled by chemotherapy for weeks, maybe months, even possibly years, I looked out of his spotless eighth-story window, across the road at a billboard featuring a sexy young woman with long naked legs and I wanted to leap through it.

Incurable cancer. I had incurable cancer. Henceforth my life would be hospitals, chemotherapy, whatever that was, doctors, tests, more tests, blood tests, scans. I would have to submit myself, my body, over and over. I was unable to grasp the full impact of what he was saying about my death, but the life he was describing seemed unbearable. The lettering above the woman on the billboard read "Live a Little." I wanted to jump.

Once, when I was a child, my brother brutalized my dolls, and so my father and I took my armless, legless, headless dolls to the doll hospital to be fixed, to be healed. I remember my excitement when we returned to bring them home. I remember looking at the other dolls on the shelves of the doll hospital, awaiting their time for healing. The doll hospital was a magical place.

I'd never been to a real hospital, except to have my babies and as a child to have my tonsils out. My stepfather was a doctor. So was my ex-husband. My few medical encounters outside the family consisted of routine gynecological check-ups, and had not been pleasant. Being a patient meant being powerless, vulnerable, humiliated. The girl on the billboard taunted me with her health, her independence, her sparkling eyes, and with the glass of bubbling champagne held in her outstretched hand. She was just a two-dimensional air-brushed photo, but she shimmered with vitality while I was being told that my life was over.

Back then in the oncologist's pristine office it wasn't the thought of death that reduced me to a puddle of grief. It was the thought of life, life as a patient, as the invalid, dehumanized recipient of a variety of "treatments." I shuddered. This was literally my worst nightmare. For most of my life, I'd thought that my unplumbed terror of medical "tests" and "treatments" had indeed been just a horrible dream, but it hadn't, unless a repressed memory can be called a horrible dream. Some years earlier, the turning point of two years of regular psychotherapy had been the recollection of a childhood episode that at the time had been too traumatic to store away for future reference. I had pushed it far, far down, down to the bottom of the pool, way beyond the reaches of my conscious mind.

The memory was triggered by a letter to the editor in Melbourne's daily newspaper, but I believe that if I was not halfway through therapy I would have read it without twigging that it was in a sense written to me. I would have continued to forget. It was from a woman who as a young girl in the 1960s had been given hormones in order to stunt her growth. In response to an article that had appeared in the paper the previous week, she wrote, "we were not 'public-spirited individuals who volunteered for treatment.' Neither we, nor our parents, ever knew that we were part of an ongoing experiment."

I read this letter sitting at my kitchen table with the newspaper spread out before me. When I read the words "ongoing experiment," the memory surfaced, not in words – in images. I recalled my nine-year-old, naked, prepubescent self standing in a room full of people, men in white coats, drawing on my skin with magic markers, measuring my bones, taking photographs of my body parts, telling me to turn, this way and that. My grandmother had brought me to this place, and she was sitting there, in the room, witnessing my humiliation. Seated at my kitchen table, as the images rose and refused to return to that safe place within, I felt something like a vise clutching my heart. I had been one of those "tall girls." Well, almost. My parents had worried about my height. I was always taller than my older brother, and I was head and shoulders above my classmates. They worried that my excessive height would lead to unhappiness in adulthood. When their GP told them about these height-stunting hormones, they took me to be tested – not to a hospital, to a university. As far as I know, those photographs are still sitting with thousands of others somewhere in the vaults of the University of Melbourne.

I "failed" the test. After being measured and photographed from every possible angle in every possible way in a room in which people, adults, men in white coats walked freely back and forth, it was decided that my projected adult height was significantly less than the minimum six foot that was required before the treatment could commence. Others were not so lucky. Their treatment brought on early puberty, weight gain, depression, and serious illnesses later in life. Throughout their treatment, they were subjected to regular measuring and photography sessions. Why? Because, said the merchants of this new miracle drug, a too-tall girl may feel embarrassed dating shorter men. Her career choices would be limited. She couldn't, for instance, become a ballet dancer or an air hostess. And this justified stunting her growth. I know this, for a fact, because after the emergence of my repressed memory I was invited to join a control group in a government-funded study into the effects of the "tall girl" episode. Still cowering before the images in my head, I declined.

Over the years that traumatic experience became jumbled in my mind with Holocaust images, particularly with what I'd heard and read and with pictures I'd seen of Nazi medical experiments on children. Around the time of my own participation in a medical experiment, I became obsessed with the Holocaust. I read everything I could find – Eli Wiesel, Primo Levi, Jerzy Kosinski, and of course Anne Frank. Despite the horror, I couldn't stop. The awful images had set up camp in my mind. They laid siege to my imagination. In my adult life I have known people who are addicted to pornography. Their addiction always reminds me of my childhood Holocaust obsession. To this day, I refuse to enter Holocaust museums that display pictures of Jews being exposed and humiliated. They infuriate me. These people never gave their permission to be photographed like that and hung upon a wall, and neither did I.

In those days of late childhood, Holocaust images came to me as I fell asleep, and at school and at home and on my way to school and on my way home, and when I watched TV and when I attended family gatherings and when I walked to and from the bus stop and when I unwrapped my sandwich at recess. Whenever. For a while I think I dwelled inside the Holocaust, in a world both nightmarish and daydreamy, in which I was always the victim, objectified, tortured, humiliated. A world filled with terror to which I was twistedly attracted. I believe that many children endure such episodes. Mine, however, became enmeshed with my "tall girl" experience.

13

Four decades after my ordeal, no longer "tall," I sat in a sterile office on the top floor of the Worthington, feeling as if I was drowning, while the nondescript oncologist wrote out my three options on a blank sheet of paper. The mastectomy was ruled out. I was too sick, and the tumors in my lungs needed urgent attention. So there it was. My first option was to do nothing, and die. Or I could give chemotherapy a go. Or I could participate in a drug trial, which, I gathered, meant being a guinea pig for some unproven treatment. He slid some pamphlets across the desk. This was unbearable. Amira helped me up and led me from the room, leaving my mother alone with the doctor. My mother told Doug later that the oncologist had gone on to say that I had stage-four metastatic breast cancer, my lungs were a mess, and he doubted I'd live out the year.

I didn't know he'd said that. Doug told me months later. Back then I was crying with Amira in the waiting room, but I knew enough to know I had entered a nightmare, and it seemed there was no way out. The oncologist, whose name I do not remember, sent me for another blood test. I could do it now, he said, on my way out, on the first floor. He booked me in for a bone scan the following day. Before he decided on a treatment he had to know the extent of the damage.

Doug was back on deck for the bone scan. Back we went to the bloody Worthington, past the spot where I'd been run over, winding with the brown Yarra River and the tanned joggers, over the bridge, to search for a parking spot near the hospital. We couldn't find a close parking spot, so Doug dropped me off at the entrance and went on to search further afield. I made my way painfully, breathlessly, to the Department of Medical Imaging. I knew my way around the Worthington by now, but the place didn't feel familiar. It would never feel familiar. It was too modern, too sterile. There were too many Rothko prints on the walls. This time, I didn't have to wait. I was ushered into a back room, injected with dye, some kind of contrast that would illuminate my bones on a scan, and told to come back, bypassing the reception and the waiting room, in four hours. By the time I returned to the front desk, Doug had arrived.

What to do for four hours? The only person I knew in this neighborhood was my psychiatrist, Dr. Birch. I called his office and miraculously there was an opening in a few hours. I hadn't seen him for months. I don't know why I hadn't thought to call him during the traumas of the past month. Why hadn't I thought of him as I sank day by day, test by test? For some reason he wasn't one of the people I'd turned to, gripped onto, begging to be saved.

Strange, when not too many years ago I couldn't imagine life without this man. I'd followed the river and crossed the bridge to see him weekly, then fortnightly, for two years, as we worked to untie the knot that I'd made of my life and delved back, way back to hazy memories, all the way back to that which was unremembered, the childhood trauma that was the key to everything.

When it emerged, triggered by the letter to the editor, I'd begged him for pills, for something to make the pain go away, and he refused, insisting I feel it, forbidding me to repress it again. I'd hated him then, but I bore the pain and came out the other side and began to heal. Some months later he'd informed me that my therapy was finished. Therapy, he said, should have a beginning, a middle, and an end. I had successfully come to the end. I could of course make an appointment to see him any time, if I felt an occasional inability to live with uncertainty. But that wouldn't be often, he said, because now I could be my own shrink. I could "check in" with myself.

But now that I had cancer I was no longer certain of anything, not the next hour, not the next breath. The uncertainty was intolerable. My body had betrayed me. I couldn't trust myself for anything anymore.

Despite all I'd revealed to him, Dr. Birch and I had always been formal with each other. I never called him by his first name. We never shook hands. A hug was out of the question, unimaginable. I'd always liked him just the way he was, distant, caring, able to withstand my occasional bouts of anger, allowing me to be the center of his universe for one hour a week, for a fixed fee.

Doug and I spent the first few hours in a bookshop that was also a café. I don't know how we managed it, but we had fun. I chose a book for each of the kids and I was delighted with the prospect of bringing something home for them, as I'd often done quite spontaneously when they were little. In this avant-garde, literary atmosphere the Worthington and the cancer seemed far away and unrelated.

We hid from the cancer behind the books, behind the coffee cups, behind our banter. We both knew it was still out there, ultimately unavoidable, but the respite, the pretense at frivolity in the warm friendly bookshop was sweet, and we relished it.

It was a chilly, blustery Melbourne day. The wind slapped me as we made for the car. I felt like a wet withering reed, trampled upon.

Whenever I'd visited Dr. Birch in the past I'd had to wait, sometimes for up to an hour. This time, just like at the Worthington, I was ushered in immediately. Doug rolled a cigarette and waited outside.

Strange, strange, strange. I glossed over the cancer, the diagnostic process, my lungs, the bone scan, chemo, just to fill him in. I didn't mention fear, panic, or dread. I decided that the real purpose of my visit that day as I waited for the contrast to make its way through my body was to talk about issues between Doug and the kids. Is that strange? He didn't act as if it was. With the exception of a few gentle grunts, he was silent and expressionless during my brief and rather emotionless cancer update. That was a relief. By then I'd already learned to be guarded when discussing it. I was so, so tired of having to take care of other people's fears. It was heartless of them really, to pour themselves out like that before me. I was overwhelmed by their tears. I had enough of my own.

While carrying on about the kids, I mentioned that Doug was waiting outside. Dr. Birch asked if we could invite him in. Sure, I said, sure.

Now it was his turn to gloss. He glossed over the issues between Doug and the kids and gently steered us back to the cancer. He wouldn't let it lurk outside. He invited it in, and embraced it. Many women who consulted him had breast cancer, he said, establishing his credentials. Would I consider adopting a vegan diet and learning to meditate?

So my formal, suit-and-tie shrink was into alternative medicine! I wasn't surprised.

Nothing really surprised me any more in those action-packed days. He recommended a book on veganism. Since my initial diagnosis four weeks earlier, I'd been preached to by scores of well-wishers pushing miracle cures ranging from holy men to apricot kernels to weird healing machines. It was confronting, and exasperating, especially when I was told that physical illness is always a symptom of spiritual sickness. What deep part of me, I was asked, had secretly wanted this illness and invited it in?

What did they know of my spiritual life? How could they be so sure? Perhaps I was like Job, tested, but not guilty. The smugness of it infuriated me. But this was different. I trusted Dr. Birch. He'd steered me through a great darkness, past and present. He and I must be about the same age. If anything, I would be older, but he's always been a kind of father figure, as a good shrink should be, I suppose.

I told him I didn't want to read the book. I would become a vegan, right now, this minute, and I would learn to meditate. At last someone I chose to believe had given me something to hold on to. Why hadn't I thought of him sooner? He told me I could continue to be in touch with him over the phone, as the journey in to see him might be too much for me in the near future. I could make an appointment with the receptionist. So he thought I had a far future! I grabbed his optimism, as if it was the last raft in an endless ocean.

I'd always loved the quiet of Dr. Birch's consulting rooms, and the way we sat opposite each other in plush leather chairs. His desk was in the corner. His books were neatly piled on the shelves. The clock was there, telling me exactly how much time was left for our session. Once or twice I'd picked up a hint of pipe tobacco. I wondered if it was his. I felt secure in there, cocooned. His voice was gentle, never overly emotive or surprised, never judgmental. Being in Dr. Birch's office was like lying on the floor of a gently rocking wooden boat on a sparkling lake on a warm spring day. Of course there had been stormy days as well, when I was stung by wind and rain, when I clung to the sides of the boat fearing it would capsize. But on that day, less than twenty-four hours after I'd been told I had incurable cancer, not knowing what torrents lay ahead, the consulting room was a refuge. I wished I could wrap myself up in it, while the storm raged outside.

Back at Worthington, at Medical Imaging, we bypassed reception and went straight to the scanning rooms. A number of patients were already there, waiting their turn for the scanner. Doug and I sat, preparing to stare blankly and listen to the tick of the clock, but a nurse appeared immediately and approached me smiling, to lead me gently by the arm into the scanning room.

And then it hit me. I was getting preferential treatment. I was too ill to be left waiting, too ill to be wasting precious time. My scan results were needed urgently. My life was hanging by a thread. I looked at the nurse's compassionate face and shook with terror.

The bone scan took a while, but by then, after a month of cancer, day in, day out, time wasn't what it used to be. Before Cancer, time was open ended, yet I felt I had to account for every minute. I had to be achieving something, preferably a number of things, every moment. The more I multitasked, the better I felt about myself. My pride in multitasking was, I think, born with motherhood, when breast-feeding with the phone wedged between ear and hunched shoulder while making a cup of tea was considered an art form. Now, lying motionless under the scanner, seeing death as my future instead of some vague immortality, I let the minutes go. I would like to keep this, I thought, this doing nothing. It took me back, way back to my childhood, to lying on my bed reading novels and eating oranges for hours upon hours, to lying on the grass, staring at the sky, to doodling in class, making patterns with the letters of my name, for no reason, not to achieve, not to accomplish. I'd forgotten what a gift it was.

I knew all about it in theory. It was the basis of most of my teaching, this nothingness, this not-doing that is the heart and soul of all creation. I spoke about it with eloquence, but it had been years since I'd allowed myself to just stop, to stop filling in time, and experience it in all its vast emptiness. I used my time to study the theory of the empty space. I made notes and prepared classes on it. Rabbi Hoffman spoke of it often, this empty space, this great black hole that holds the world in place. He called it Shabbat, the holy Sabbath, the day for being, not for doing. Shabbat, he said, was the still point at the very heart of the busy days of the whirling week. I listened, I nodded, but even on the Sabbath when I neither drove nor wrote I had devoted myself to reading, learning, achieving.

My teacher Avivah Zornberg, quoting Keats and then Marion Milner, calls not-doing "diligent indolence" and "doodle time." From her I learned that it needs to be learned, or perhaps relearned, and cherished.

So this is what she means, I thought. This is doing nothing. And lying there being scanned, with the death sentence of advanced cancer upon me, I smiled.

The bone scan was clear, the first bit of good news in weeks. Now I needed to start treatment. At night in the dark, the oncologist's words pierced me. I imagined being shut up in a casket, bereft of air and light, being lowered into the ground and covered with dirt. No! It was unbearable. I wept and prayed for mercy.

"You have kept count of my wanderings. Put my tears in Your bottle: they are already in Your book."

Doug held me. "The man is an idiot," he whispered. "By what crystal ball does he decide how long you live? You can't let him treat you. We'll find someone else."

I had to agree. The thought of going back to that sterile office, or to anywhere else in the bloody Worthington, set my teeth on edge.

14

We decided to look for a woman oncologist who worked on our side of town. We asked all our medically connected friends, and one name kept reappearing, a very well-known oncologist, famous really. I was warned, though, that like all top-echelon specialists she was not very available. I called her office and was told she had no free appointments for weeks. I begged. Have your scans sent over, said the receptionist, and I'll make sure the doctor sees them. I arranged for the Worthington doomsayer to send the scans across. The following day the receptionist called.

"The doctor says you need immediate treatment. Your situation is urgent. You can't afford to wait. Find someone else."

I was devastated. I called a doctor friend, who spent the morning asking around and following leads. He called back with the name of a woman oncologist attached to St. Katherine's Hospital, which was just down the road from us. He said she was highly recommended, though not as famous as the oncologist who'd been booked solid.

I called her office and explained the situation. The receptionist told me to have the scans sent across now, and to come in the morning, at 8 a.m. The doctor would come in early, she said, and see me before her day began.

She made the appointment without even asking the doctor. That was right. That was what a caring medical professional should do. Thus began our relationship with Lara.

St. Katherine's Hospital is set in a leafy, middle-class neighborhood. It's only four stories high and the consulting rooms are on the ground floor. I didn't have to think about jumping any more. St. Katherine's has many outdoor settings, little courtyards with wooden benches set among flowering trees. It's peaceful. There are no Rothkos on the walls, just pictures of people who work there – doctors, nurses, technicians, volunteers, cleaners. The staff seem happy. When I'm there I have a sense of people working together. It's very reassuring. St. Katherine's is a Catholic hospital, founded by a saint whose picture is ubiquitous in the wards. At Christmas time carols filter gently through the PA system and large, detailed Nativity scenes are displayed at both main entrances.

Well, I thought, as Doug and I made our way to Lara's office, I'd rather be in a place of faith, any faith, than in a place of no faith at all. I had to concede that every hospital is a place of faith, but most place their faith exclusively in science, in the absolute power of the human mind. This often leaves no space for faith in the individual as the bearer of a unique spirit, or perhaps a soul, with its own unique destiny. Without faith in our individuality, we become statistics, numbers, prognoses.

During my month of diagnosis, I'd been told a number of times that cancer is not really separable from the person it invades. It manifests in each individual differently and unpredictably, and this is why it is so difficult to find a cure. In other words, we all have our own stories, and in truth a "prognosis" is nothing but assumption and hubris. Statistics are meaningless when it comes to the individual.

At St. Katherine's I felt like an individual. I was living out my own story, which was different from every other person's story. I was not a statistic. My prognosis was no different from that of all life on earth. My life would end in death.

Directly after my initial diagnosis of early breast cancer, I was repeatedly asked "What's your prognosis?" Even more than depressing me, the question annoyed me. Once, in exasperation, I responded, "I don't know. What's yours?"

After a shocked silence the inquirer said indignantly, "But I'm not sick!"

"Maybe not," I cruelly replied, "but you and I are going to die, on a particular date, at a particular hour of the day. What's yours?"

The move back across town to St. Katherine's, just down the road, felt right. I still lived in constant terror of the shadow of death, but a little bit of light had begun to creep in.

Lara is a young woman – well, younger than I – a sweet, petite woman with a girl's voice and a warm smile. At that first meeting she didn't waste any time telling me that I was going to die. She quietly explained that a mastectomy would not be advisable at this point. I'd need to start chemo straight away. For the first time, we got an intelligible description of "chemo" and of general side effects like fatigue and nausea.

Lara doesn't scare me with horror stories or gruesome scenarios. She doesn't address what "could happen," as it hasn't yet happened, and if it does, then she'll explain it and we'll deal with it. I like that approach. It suits me. Back then, four weeks into cancer, I'd already learned not to google. Googling "advanced or metastatic breast cancer" was like being forced to watch oneself being sentenced to a slow and tortured death. Investigative Internet sessions always ended in fears and tears. I was committed to cease doing that to myself.

All I knew was that I was to have a series of weekly intravenous chemo sessions, that I'd need to take pre-meds – steroids – that I'd start on Monday, and that Lara would visit me at Day Oncology to see that everything went smoothly.

Looking back over the past two and a half years, at the anaphylactic attack, the crippling nausea, the overwhelming fatigue, the cracked nails, the hair loss, the menopause, the depression, I am grateful to Lara for not going into detail. She just guided us to the next step. I knew, vaguely, that it could be much, much worse, but I prayed that I would never have to find out. Lara allowed me to learn at my own pace, to become a seasoned cancer patient through experience. As I slowly learned, she slowly became more open with me, calling chemo "cruel and unusual punishment," smiling her broad smile when scan results were good and rejoicing with us when they were good enough for a chemo break. And when the news was not so good, meaning when it was bad, she helped us move on, step by step, discussing the options. Even when the cancer broke through the blood-brain barrier and entered my head, she didn't talk about prognoses and drug trials. For a science-oriented, left-brain kind of woman, she is wonderfully open to possibility, including the possibility of a miracle. I think we work well together.

We had the weekend to prepare for chemo. I felt like a child about to start at a new school. Day Oncology. It sounded like a new school for toddlers.

Early on Monday morning I staggered, heavily supported by Doug, down a long corridor, to Day Oncology. What now is a part of my life was then so new, so frightening. My Day Oncology experiences over the past few years have been overwhelmingly positive, but as luck or whoever would have it, on that first morning we scored an odd-mannered nurse, strangely unmoved by my plight. She seemed very distracted. When she had me seated, she asserted that I was there for a bone biopsy.

Doug and I had no idea what she was talking about, but the flagrant error made us nervous, very nervous. She rechecked the records, discovered that I was there for chemo, and returned to apologize, but she still seemed elsewhere, not at all present. She left mid-morning. I was told she was unwell, and in our many visits since that morning we have never seen her again.

These days, I know most of the nurses, some quite well. The other patients are usually pleasant, quiet. We are seated in rows of specially designed recliner chairs. Sometimes we chat with our neighbors, but not often. We read, talk to the nurses, or to the person who accompanied us. If we suffer, we do it quietly. But on the morning of my true initiation into the world of cancer, the woman seated opposite me became hysterical and had to be sedated. She hadn't yet started her chemo session. The hysteria happened when the nurses tried to insert a drip by way of a needle in the back of her hand. She was too distressed to stay still long enough for the nurses to find a vein. I was waiting for my designated nurse, who as I mentioned seemed a little whacky, to connect me to my drip. The woman's hysteria filled me with horror. The unspeakable kind of horror. I looked mutely at Doug and he squeezed my hand. I never again saw anyone respond to a needle as that woman did, but back then I thought it must be a regular occurrence.

It takes fortitude to endure the chemo needle. Some people opt for a "port," a semi-permanent pathway to a vein, but after watching one woman brought in screaming from the pain of an infected port I've staunchly stuck to the needle in the back of the hand. Apparently my veins are "fine" and hard to pinpoint, and at times it takes a while to locate a suitable one. Early on, in one of our telephone appointments, Dr. Birch taught me "yoga breathing." In for five, hold it for two, out for five, hold it for two, and so on. I find it remarkably effective, especially when I close my eyes as well. I'm often told how "brave" I am. I don't feel brave. I usually feel more like a powerless victim of circumstance. But when I do my yoga breathing and hold my hand perfectly still and relaxed for the needle, I feel incredibly brave.

I wish I'd learned that technique much earlier in life. It might have served me well in the bomb shelter in Safed. I'd often tried to mask my panic, but I'd never understood that panic wasn't necessary, or helpful. I'd panicked over the craziest things: running late for an appointment, losing my way in the car, a broken appliance, a child a few minutes late home from school. I was a worrier. My worries wouldn't let me sleep. Had I paid the electricity bill? Had I been unwittingly offensive in a conversation that day? Had I locked the door before I went to bed? I suppose worrying is a cousin, a few times removed, of panic.

I panicked too easily. Perhaps that was why Rabbi Hoffman had challenged me to return to Safed. He needn't have bothered. Safed had come to me.

The first chemo session was long – eight hours – a whole working day in the chair. I was given the Herceptin first, then the Taxol, both administered very slowly, in case I reacted.

I was high on steroids, grinning inappropriately and feeling overactive. I felt awful, restless, spacey, trapped. Being pinned to a chair, high on steroids, while poison is introduced into one's system is no cup of tea. A few seem to take it in their stride, but I doubt I ever will. I can handle targeted therapies, but when it comes to chemo, which attacks all my cells, good and bad, I suffer.

The treatment was to continue for eight consecutive weeks. On the second week, I had an anaphylactic attack. I'd never heard of it either. It means "life threatening allergic reaction." Apparently I was allergic to Taxol. I'm not the allergic type. My only known allergy until then was to bee stings, and I'd avoided them for decades, so when I suddenly felt like an over-inflated balloon and had difficulty breathing, I had no idea what was going on. Of course I panicked. I remember the tap on the drip being closed, and my chair being yanked back into full recline. I remember lips on my ear, whispered words echoing strangely in my eardrum. "You're okay. It's all right. Relax." It could have been an angel, or a nurse. Months later, Doug told me it was him. It was a wonderfully affirming voice. A voice of life.

Lara was summoned and the chemo session was cut short. I was given the anti-anxiety drug Ativan, a blessing hitherto unknown to me. It made me feel wonderfully light, buoyant, unable to sink. Ativan has since seen me through a number of murky moments. When I came back to earth, I was upset about missing out on the chemo. How would it affect my chances? A friend involved in cancer research pointed out that if I reacted that strongly to Taxol, even a third of a dose must have knocked out armies of cancer cells. I don't know if there's any truth in that, but it sounded logical, and I decided to believe him.

After the anaphylactic episode, I switched to Taxotere, a synthetic form of Taxol, which is derived from the bark of the yew tree, and continued for another six weekly sessions. The side effects were cumulative, severe in the beginning and unbearable by the end. Nausea, fatigue, chest pain. No hair loss, however. I learned then that fatigue doesn't mean "very tired." One evening, when Doug was out, I was sitting in bed, propped by pillows, and couldn't muster the energy to lie down. The fatigue had paralyzed me. I couldn't move my hand to turn on the bedside light. I couldn't use my voice to call out to one of the kids. I sat there for three hours, staring helplessly into the darkened room, until Doug arrived. That, I learned, is fatigue.

Every day of those first eight weeks of chemo was a storm to be endured. By day I lay exhausted in a recliner chair in the kitchen, and by night I lay next to Doug, trying to will the thought of burial out of my mind. Back then, death, and specifically burial, was my greatest fear. This sudden knowledge of my mortality caused me unimaginable terror. What if a dead person still had some kind of consciousness? There's no way of knowing, unless you believe in ghosts. Near-death experiences don't count, because none of them experienced being buried. As a Jew, I am destined for burial, not cremation. I lay in bed trying to escape the thought of being enclosed in a coffin, lowered into a pit, hearing the spadefuls of dirt separate me forever from sensing and being sensed. I was very afraid. I couldn't lie in absolute darkness. We kept the bathroom light on so that a crack was visible under the door.

I don't feel that way anymore. Somewhere in one of my alternative-health forays, I heard that absolute darkness at night helps the body to produce melatonin, and that melatonin fights cancer cells. I turned off the bathroom light, and a strange thing happened. I learned to love the dark, as I had as a child. These days I feel embraced by it. Sometimes at night I will enter an utterly dark room, just to stand in it, to feel so utterly at one with my environment, safe and unobserved.

15

Every week of that first round of chemo brought new challenges. A month earlier, when I was first diagnosed, I'd canceled all my speaking engagements and stopped teaching. Soon after I started chemo, however, I decided to reinstate one weekly class, on Thursday mornings, from my home. Somehow it felt easier to face people from behind a teacher's desk, and to speak of my experiences through the prism of Torah.

The world as I knew it, all my frames of reference, had disappeared. My new world was not yet familiar, and my sense of myself in it was still very shaky. Most one-on-one interactions had not been working for me. I either felt preached to, or totally misunderstood. Very few of my acquaintances knew the difference between early and advanced breast cancer, and I resented having to be the one to explain it, not once, but over and over, often to the same person. No, I will never finish treatment. No, I will not be cured unless they find a cure, or I become the lucky recipient of a miracle. Yes, I know that such-and-such had a mastectomy thirty years ago and is still going strong. Yes, she's a survivor. No, I wanted to shout, that does not give me hope. It makes me depressed. I felt like Job surrounded by false comforters. Why couldn't they understand? Looking back, I can see that I did not yet understand myself. I didn't know how to be Debbie-with-incurable-cancer because I didn't yet fully inhabit her.

I was nervous before the first Thursday morning class. These were people I'd known and studied with for years. How would they treat me? Would I be faced with a roomful of pitying eyes, or worse still, tears? Perhaps no one would be able to meet my eye.

Perhaps no one would show up. In the minutes before the first students arrived I was convinced that this had been a crazy idea.

I teach in our front room, which I suppose in our hundred-year-old home was once called "the parlor." It's a beautiful room, very large, with ornate cornices and light fittings, a mantelpiece and fireplace and windows facing the front garden. As my teaching room, it is furnished with five trestle tables set up in a U shape, with my teaching table, in front of the mantelpiece, placed in the gap of the U. The carpet is a plush burnt orange, and with the help of my friend Chooch I'd chosen an Indian-looking material that picked up the same burnt orange for the tablecloths. On the walls are five large framed prints, one for each of the Five Books of Moses, a gift from my artist friend Victor Majzner. It is a beautiful room, especially in the morning, when the sun filters through the trees and shines through the windows. On these sunny mornings, my teaching room glows.

When I teach, I leave the front door unlocked, and tea, coffee, and a boiling urn in the kitchen. That morning, about fifteen minutes before the class was due to begin, people started trickling in. A little later they were flowing through the door. I shouldn't have worried. It was wonderful. It felt like a reunion, a celebration, an affirmation. When there was no more room at the tables, people seated themselves in the adjoining dining room. I did not feel pitied, or judged. The room was full of love, glowing with it, and I was filled with gratitude.

For a number of years I'd taught the weekly Torah reading in that room, to these people, on Thursday mornings. We'd study the passage that was being read that week in the synagogue, looking at ancient, medieval, and modern commentaries. Week by week, we worked our way through the Five Books of Moses, and when we finished, we'd begin again. There was always something new to learn, a new perspective, an alternative view to discover. Studying Torah is a bit like standing on a mountain peak on a clear day, on a cloudy day, on a rainy day, in a storm. It's like beating a track through heavy jungle, and like wandering in a rainforest and traversing a desert and living in New York City. My readings were always illuminated by whatever was going on in my life at that time. I couldn't help reading Torah that way. Even when I'd read it as the "Old Testament" at my Church of England primary school, the text had been alive for me, infinitely evocative. I'd always read it as my story, and I'd always known that my story was intimately entwined with others, like a wild vine, ultimately unravelable.

When I rediscovered the "Old Testament" as "Torah," as the bedrock of my people, I knew that I had always known it, in all its infinite variety. It had always been engraved within me, and every new discovery, each new delight, was really an unveiling. The Midrash teaches that each of us knows the entire Torah in utero, and we forget it during the trauma of birth. Each time we learn something new, when we are amazed by what we learn, we are actually remembering something forgotten long, long ago.

When I had received the first cancer diagnosis, my Thursday morning group had just begun the Book of Numbers. When I resumed teaching eight weeks later we were entering Deuteronomy, the last of the Five Books.

In the interim, it was Torah that sustained me. I suppose the threat of imminent death can throw a person either way. Atheists hanging by their fingernails from the sides of jagged cliffs may experience an overwhelming desire to make promises to a god in whom they have never believed. And among the pious, those who believe that religious devotion is rewarded in this world may lose their faith with a sudden reversal of good fortune. At times I have fallen into both categories. I think that most of us would have to agree that life is not fair. Bad things can happen to good people, suddenly, inexplicably, cruelly. Children starve, women are raped, whole populations are wiped out, not because each one of them sinned and was condemned to a horrible death by some great and terrible deity. I don't believe in that vengeful god, and yet I can't not believe in the holiness that vivifies this world, both in its sunlit places and in its terrifying shadows.

My years of study of the Warsaw Ghetto writings of the Rebbe of Piacezna served me well when I found myself trapped by cancer. The year before, when Katyusha rockets fell on the sleepy town of Safed, I fled. If I could flee from cancer now, I would. But I can't. Those first weeks after the final, terrible diagnosis, I begged, I prayed real prayer, tearful prayers from the heart, the broken, desperate heart. I was groping in the dark, facing the cool slime at the bottom of the pool, when my Rebbe, the holy Rebbe of Piacezna who was murdered by the Nazis in November 1943, reached out, all the way from the Garden of Eden, and saved me.

It's written in the Talmud that if anyone recites the words of a dead scholar, the lips of that scholar mutter in the grave. The Rebbe of Piacezna quoted this Talmudic teaching in the *Eish Kodesh*, his text from the Warsaw Ghetto, and whenever I read these words, I feel them to be true. I hear him speak directly to me.

It must have been shortly after I returned home from the lung biopsy, when I was struggling to come to terms with the words "incurable" and "terminal." Rabbi Hoffman called. We'd continued to have brief telephone conversations, but we hadn't studied together since the session during which the breast-screen clinic had called to ask me back for more tests.

I was alone in my room. The door was closed. When Rabbi Hoffman called I felt free to pour out my heart.

"What's happening?" I asked him tearily. "What's happening to me?"

The "why's" wouldn't arise until much later. Those first weeks, I struggled desperately with the "what" – I just couldn't fathom what was happening, what had happened to my world.

Rabbi Hoffman responded with what I thought were platitudes. He assured me that despite everything, despite the grim biopsy results…who knows? Who knows what could happen?

I felt angry and unheard. Then he cajoled me into studying some *Eish Kodesh* with him. It was the week of the Torah portion in which Moses sends out spies to scout the Promised Land. They return with fearful tales of cruel giants and highly fortified cities. The place was impossible to conquer, they said. They tried to persuade the Israelites to return to Egypt, for surely slavery would be preferable to what awaited them in this "Promised Land."

Two of the twelve spies, Joshua and Caleb, dissented and urged the people to have faith and keep going. Neither Rabbi Hoffman nor I could recall what the Piacezna Rebbe had written about this episode. We looked it up – Rabbi Hoffman in his home in Denver, Colorado, and I in my Melbourne sickbed – sixty-seven years after it was originally written in unimaginable, overwhelming, and hopeless conditions. It was a very short piece, just three paragraphs. We found that in the Warsaw Ghetto in June 1940, the Rebbe had noted that Caleb did not try to persuade the people to keep going by demolishing the arguments of the others. He didn't dispute their reports of fearsome giants and the great likelihood of defeat. He simply said, "We must go forth."

Rabbi Hoffman asked if I had the strength to read. I wasn't sure, but I knew that back then, in the Warsaw Ghetto in June 1940, the Rebbe hadn't had the strength to write.

"Yes," I said, and I read aloud, as best I could, over the phone. I read, and as I read, we both gasped. The Rebbe's lips were moving! He was speaking to me! He was answering me.

I read: "Not only when we see reasonable openings and paths for our salvation to occur within the laws of nature must we have faith that God will save us, and take heart, but also, when we see no way for salvation to come through natural means, we must still believe…. A person needs to say, 'Yes, all the logic and facts may indeed be true. The people who inhabit the land may be very strong, and their cities well fortified, and so forth, but I still believe in God, Who is beyond any boundaries, and above all nature. I believe that He will save us.'"

It was a straightforward statement of faith, and it was what I needed to hear. Later, by 1942, when his world was buried in a darkness hitherto unexperienced, the Rebbe's revelations were profoundly subtle, and incredibly beautiful. But on that day, at that moment, I needed to hear a proclamation of faith in a power that transcends diagnosis, prognosis, statistics. I needed to be reminded of the power of possibility, and that truly, anything could happen. By the time I finished reading, I was weeping cool, cool tears of purest joy.

The Rebbe stayed with me. Some weeks later, I was on the phone with Dr. Birch, still struggling to come to terms with my situation. He was trying to convince me that metastatic cancer is not necessarily a sudden death sentence, that in some cases it is managed for years, like a chronic disease.

"Will I have a normal lifespan?" I asked, pathetically, as if he had the power to grant me one.

"Well," he gently replied, "it's not probable, but it's possible."

Those words struck a very deep chord. The Piacezna Rebbe was still working his holy magic. My teacher Avivah Zornberg has written and spoken many powerful words, but for me the greatest of all is something she once said during an interview for a PBS radio show in America. At the burning bush, when Moses asked God to describe Himself, God replied, "I am what I am, and I will be what I will be." Avivah interpreted this to mean, "I am the very principle of becoming, of allowing the possible to happen."

Finally, some kind of peace, some sense of hope and faith fluttered within me. Nan, my meditation teacher, had instructed me to find a phrase, a sentence that could serve me as my mantra. I'd been searching for weeks, and now I had it. The Piacezna Rebbe had given it to me, through his writings, through Rabbi Hoffman, through Dr. Birch, through Avivah. Every day, for over a year, I sat quietly, alone, eyes closed, and whispered my mantra, instilling it into me, into my belief system.

"I believe with perfect faith in the principle of becoming, of allowing the possible to happen."

When my mantra hovered naturally on my lips, I returned to teaching.

I'd always read the Torah through the lens of myself or of my experiences. But when I resumed teaching that radiant Thursday morning in July, under the shadow of my stage-four cancer diagnosis, all my points of reference, the specifics of my own personal world, had disappeared. I had lost myself. All I had, all I was, was my desire to live, to hold my as yet unconceived grandchildren. I had my desire to allow the possible to happen. Nothing else mattered anymore. How could it?

This, I discovered, this nowhereness, this nothingness of pure desire, was an astonishing place from which to teach Torah.

The Book of Deuteronomy culminates in the death of Moses, whose only desire is to enter the Promised Land along with his people. He dies instead on Mt. Nebo, in the land of Moab, his wish unfulfilled. To this day, says the text, no one knows where he is buried. The death of Moses was a private, intimate interaction between the prophet and his beloved God, and so it remains. The Talmud speaks of his unmarked grave as a mysterious fulcrum, a well of desire to which lost souls are drawn, and where, in their exile, they find some comfort.

The Book of Deuteronomy contains large sections of law, but it is permeated with the prophet's longing. "Let me cross over and see that good land that is on the other side of the Jordan," he pleads, and God directs him to the peak from which to view the object of his desire. "From a distance you shall see," says God, "but you shall not enter there."

As I taught Deuteronomy and struggled through that first bout of chemo, I came closer than I ever had before to entering into the great drama of the prophet-poet who in Egypt could only stutter, the man who led his people out of slavery and through a lifetime of wilderness, who gazed with pleading eyes at that good land, but was not permitted to step across. That year I came close to understanding the Moses of Deuteronomy as a man of pure, distilled desire, a beacon of longing. I came close, but I did not cross over. I felt nauseous and tired. My bones ached. My chest heaved. Some weeks I saw people straining to hear me, because my voice was so weak. Later I was told that these were among the most potent, most articulate classes I'd ever given, that after them people stepped out into the rest of their Thursdays as if into a strange world, that their inner worlds remained with Moses on the steppes of Moab.

For my part, these were among the most rewarding classes I'd ever taught. The sense of having communicated, really communicated, was precious beyond measure. The rest of the week I was mostly curled up in a ball of suffering and self-pity. I was often surrounded by loving, well-meaning friends and family, but it was as if there was a wall between us. Except for Doug, no one seemed to understand. On Thursdays, when I sat with my students in the sunlit, burnt-orange front room, I felt swaddled in love. In that space my heart and my lips were circumcised. I was exhausted afterwards, but those classes saved me from the pit, they filled my home with hope. After class, a few of us would gather in the kitchen. I'd collapse into my recliner chair, sip tea, and listen to the conversation flow like living water through my home.

16

There were other moments of respite during those chemo weeks. My ongoing correspondence with Avivah Zornberg was another jewel in my week. She was far away in Jerusalem, yet I felt closer to her than to many of the people around me. Very early in our relationship she had called me her "ideal reader," and now, after years of sharing, I think we both knew that this was reciprocal. We corresponded in what to others must surely look like some kind of code language. Our minds were tuned to the same wavelength. Often just a word, an image, could convey an entire conversation. Avivah had been at the other end of the computer throughout the ordeal of my diagnosis, and she was with me during those eight weeks of chemo, eight weeks of Deuteronomy, sharing her thoughts, listening appreciatively to mine. I felt blessed by the good fortune of her friendship.

I continued to speak with Rabbi Hoffman on the phone; he continued to find ways to boost my spirits, but now I was trying to do the same for him. One of his sons had been involved in a horrific car accident that had left him a quadriplegic. How suddenly our worlds transform. As he lived every parent's nightmare, Rabbi Hoffman proved to me that we could emulate the Rebbe of Piacezna, we could find ways to respond to the darkness. We didn't have to drown. A few months later, Chana, my former landlady in Safed, was diagnosed with uterine cancer. Chana had remained in Safed throughout the Second Lebanon War, during which the ancient Galilean city was repeatedly attacked. After the war she compiled a book of essays and letters written by residents during the crisis. It was published under the title *Faith Under Fire*. By any standard, I considered her a very brave woman. She never lost her faith.

She fought her cancer. She's still fighting it.

Chana, Rabbi Hoffman, and I were reunited in the bomb shelter, and this time I had no option but to stay with them, and be still.

By the eighth week of chemo I felt I'd reached the end of my resources. I didn't care about the consequences. I couldn't take any more. With the exception of the time I spent with Moses and the troupe on the plains of Moab on Thursday mornings, I was barely functioning. I needed a break. My only joy was the insensibility of sleep. What good was this treatment, if it stripped me of almost every earthly pleasure? When we'd begun, Lara had said that I'd be having sixteen rounds of chemo, with scans mid-way to see how I was going. Somehow in my mind I'd translated that into eight weeks, followed by a break. After the scans, I turned up with Doug at her office, ready to demand some relief. Lara was beaming. My scan results were great. The two main lesions on my lungs had shrunk considerably. One breast tumor could no longer be detected and the other was a third its original size. In the hope of maintaining this welcome turn of events, I would have to remain on Herceptin, which would mean a visit to Day Oncology every three weeks, but no more Taxotere! Herceptin, a "targeted chemo," had minimal side effects. No more Taxotere meant no more living hell. Lara was happy, we were happy, but it was only when I saw the reaction of our medically informed friends that I realized just how happy we should be. Some time later, Lara told me that if I hadn't responded to those first rounds of chemo, my prospects would have been pretty grim.

One of the lessons of advanced cancer is that the reprieves are conditional. There's always something else to worry about. As well as showing that the two tumors originally detected on my lungs had shrunk considerably, the latest scans showed hitherto undetected tiny dots on both lungs, lots of dots, lots and lots, way too many to count. They hadn't been detected on the scans that were done before I started treatment, because they had been hidden by the fluid on my lungs. Lara was puzzled. We could be looking at scar tissue from some earlier illness. Or these could be tiny spots of metastasized cancer. We wouldn't know until the next set of scans, three months later. If they all remained unchanged, they were probably due to scarring. If any of them changed – either grew bigger or disappeared – then we were dealing with cancer. I thought of the drawing books I'd so loved as a child, the ones with pages of numbered dots. When you connected the dots, the picture was revealed.

"What would happen if they all got bigger?" I asked Lara.

Her smile looked more like a grimace. "It's probably scar tissue," she said. "Let's hope for that."

The thought of all those dots in my lungs expanding until they were all connected, until there was no more lung, haunted me for many months to come.

Until my cancer I'd had passing fears of illness, like other people, I suppose, but never had I been stalked by the fear of a gruesome death. Now, whenever I turned around, there it was, just behind my shoulder.

I had to learn how to live with fear. For the moment, things were good. The chemo had reduced the cancer to manageable proportions. For the moment, my life was not hanging in the balance. Yes, I had incurable cancer, but right now it was not endangering my life. Yes, I had to show up at Day Oncology every three weeks for an infusion of Herceptin. Yes, I would need to take the estrogen suppressor Tamoxifen. Yes, Tamoxifen could cause uterine cancer and Herceptin could lead to heart failure. Yes, I would need to have more scans in three months, and by then of course the picture could be entirely different, but that was not happening now.

For years, I'd read about "living in the moment" and "the power of now." I remember how impressed I was the first time I heard the adage: "Yesterday is history, tomorrow's a mystery, today is a gift and that's why we call it the present." The problem with these slogans was that when I'd needed them most, they'd failed me. When it seemed that the world had stopped spinning because a man had treated me badly, or one of my children was in trouble at school, or I received another impersonal rejection from another publisher, I didn't want to "be in the now." I wanted to be anywhere but "right here, right now." When life was good, when I was in love, when the world was in love with me, the slogans worked just fine. Where else would I want to be?

I understood the theory. Intellectually, I fathomed enough of the concept of being utterly present in the midst of utmost darkness to be able to teach it effectively, but I just couldn't achieve it, or anything like it, in practice. When my life seemed "over" because of one of a variety of disasters, I couldn't be still and allow the experience to happen. I ran around like a headless chicken, begging to be saved, to be pulled out from under the car, to be brought up from the bottom of the pool. When my repressed childhood memory had emerged, I'd begged Dr. Birch to medicate me, to make the pain go away. Now, if I wanted any kind of life at all – any *quality* of life – the hysterical response was not an option. I no longer enjoyed that luxury. The future was dark as a grave, and if I chose to dwell there, I might as well have lain down in it and died. Right now the cancer was under control. My life was not going to wait for me. I had to learn how to live now. It didn't matter that this was always the truth, that it's true for every person on the planet. Until I was literally robbed of any certainty in the future, however false that certainty might have been, I just didn't understand the meaning of being "present."

When I was given my first reprieve after those eight miserable weeks of Taxotere, I still didn't quite get it. I didn't yet have the big picture, and I hope I still don't. Even amongst those with advanced breast cancer, there are the fortunate and the not so fortunate. I didn't fully fathom back then just how fortunate I was to have received this reprieve, nor did I fully understand that its lasting forever was highly improbable. I was still too busy feeling sorry for myself. This was really the first chance I'd had to breathe since the initial diagnosis, and the whole ordeal was still too close and too traumatic to process. I was given books about other people's cancer stories, and I couldn't read them, nor could I imagine writing my own story. The Tamoxifen, the regular Herceptin infusions, the long- and short-term side effects, and especially the specter of the next set of scans, were too overwhelming. It was a relief to be off chemo, but I was still suffering its effects. I just didn't know how to relish the moment. There were too many distressing possibilities to worry about. I had to learn, and in these matters I am a slow learner.

I stuck to my vegan diet. I started daily Tai Chi practice. I meditated. I started seeing a hypnotherapist. Doug and I began to take weekends away in the country, lovely retreats to the mountains. We went for walks, and wandered around little country towns.

I began a practice I had avoided for most of my life. I made regular visits to the *mikveh*, the ritual bath. I may have gone in gratitude for not having become menopausal through chemo, as predicted. I may have gone in gratitude for not losing my hair. I may have gone to beg and rail at God. Whatever the initial motivation, I grew to love this monthly ritual immersion, especially being left alone as the living waters soaked into my skin, as my pores drank in a holiness and a healing that my mind could never fathom.

And I continued to teach.

Truth is, I was learning, slowly. Of course, I thought I'd "got it" all. And of course I became a bit of a crusader, preaching my newfound enlightenment to others. Not that I didn't literally quake with fear when the time came for my next set of scans. Sitting with Doug outside Lara's office waiting to hear the results, watching the big wall clock, tick-tock, tick-tock, reduced me to a mess of quivering nerves. I later heard this state aptly called "scanxiety." I was once more the accused, awaiting sentence.

Three months into my reprieve, things were still good. I could continue without chemo. There had been only a minimal increase in the lung and breast lesions. The dots were still there, unchanged. Once I had the scan results, I could resume breathing and return to my regimen.

I think I thought that a regimen would protect me. A daily routine of Tai Chi, protein shake, super-antioxidant blueberries, prayer and meditation created some sort of framework, woven like a bird's nest to save me from falling until I learned how to fly. Routine has always been a comfort to me. I suppose it's a great way to avoid being "present," but that doesn't prejudice me against it. My need for such comfort is too ingrained.

My daily regimen supported me through some very difficult and confronting experiences during that year of chemo reprieve. If I started the day in a regimented way, I was more able to see it through to the evening with some sort of equanimity.

I suppose it's natural that as I slowly came to terms with my own cancer, I became close to others who were more or less in the same boat. At that time I had a great, a burning desire to find someone "exactly" like me, someone who was living with metastatic breast cancer. I'd heard the stories of many, many women who had survived early breast cancer, but the only advanced cases I'd heard about were those I'd read of in the newspaper, and of course they were only newsworthy if they were famous and died of the disease. All those "lost her battle with cancer" stories didn't do much for my mindset. Now my knowledge of these things is much greater, but back then I despaired of ever meeting anyone like me, and I dismally concluded that the others were all dead. All of which, of course, served to further persuade me that I did not have long to live.

One day, I was sharing this despair with a student, a kind and sympathetic Christian, when I had a sort of epiphany. I couldn't find this woman whose survival was going to give me hope because she was me! I *was* that woman. Years from now, other women would come to me, desperate for reassurance, and I would give them hope. Now *that* was a comforting thought. I held onto it. Somewhere in the recesses of my mind, I'm still holding onto it.

I've since met women with diagnoses similar to my own, and I know that we can live with this disease, but back then, when I couldn't find anyone "just like me," I became closely connected to others in dire circumstances. Two people in particular entered my orbit – no, they broke through to my heart.

One advantage of dealing with life-threatening illness is that it makes one more qualified and more able to relate to others in similar situations. So when people with whom I really only had a passing acquaintance became seriously ill, I didn't just pay a sympathetic visit or perhaps send a card or flowers. I gravitated toward them as if we belonged with each other.

First, there was Ben. Ben had owned a flower shop, the "Garden of Eden," and I knew him as a colorful neighborhood character, a bit of a flirt, with a cowboy hat and a dazzling smile. I'd heard that he'd had cancer, and that he'd gone into remission. In our tight-knit Jewish neighborhood, one tends to hear anything that's newsworthy, eventually. I don't know when Ben started coming to my weekly classes. I just remember him appearing, often a few minutes late, with flowers, always with flowers. Not just flowers: beautiful, tender flowers, flowers that could have been hand-picked in the Garden of Eden. He would creep into the kitchen, arrange them in a vase, then settle himself quietly in the back of the room where I was teaching.

He was thinner than I remembered, but otherwise the same good-looking guy with the cheeky smile with whom I'd had a nodding acquaintance for years. I didn't know much about him apart from what I'd heard about his illness, and my perception of him as a rebellious, attractively screwed-up child of Holocaust survivors. There's a handful of middle-aged single men like him in our community, men who are attractive and exciting enough to get away with behaving like boys. As far as I know, all of them are children of survivors, and most were sent by their secular parents to Yeshiva College, our local ultra-religious Jewish boys' school. All of them rebelled, turning to sex, drugs, and alcohol in varying degrees, and all of them retained their deep ties to Jewish heritage and practice.

I didn't know why Ben was coming to my classes, but I was glad. I liked his smile. I was touched by the flowers. I liked his presence. I don't remember when he told me that he'd had a recurrence of his cancer, but it must have been soon after he first appeared in my home. Ben had pancreatic cancer. Deadly. I didn't know then that his five-year remission had been a miracle, but I've since had this confirmed for me by a number of doctors.

During the weeks and months that followed, Ben and I became very close. Although I hadn't known him well before, friends of longer standing said he was a changed man, and even I could sense some sort of shift in him. I no longer perceived him as one of the group of middle-aged Yeshiva "bad boys." Ben seemed to have undergone a major transformation. The more I got to know him, the more I could see that he didn't have to work at being the decent, loving, generous person that he had become. There was nothing superficial about his goodness. It came naturally; it sort of poured through him and out into the world like a gentle rain from heaven. He moved through life like a river winding through a landscape. I always knew when he had preceded me at Day Oncology. It was easy to tell the difference between the ordinary, slightly wilting everyday flowers that usually stood on the reception desk and the flowers that Ben brought when he came for a treatment. All the nurses loved him.

As the weeks progressed, I watched Ben weaken. Well, I watched his body weaken. His spirit was the strongest I have ever encountered. I was in awe of his courage and his capacity for suffering. When conventional chemo failed, he tried an experimental oral drug. After suffering horrendous side effects in silence for over a week, he dragged himself to his GP, who immediately called for an ambulance. When I subsequently visited him in hospital, he couldn't speak. His mouth was covered, inside and out, with abscesses. But he could still try to smile. He took my hand and pressed it. When I returned a few days later, he insisted on donning his dressing gown, shuffling to his neighbor in the next room, and struggling back with a chair for me. We sat together at his window looking out over the suburbs all the way to the Dandenong Ranges. Ben told me that he left the curtains open at night so that he would be woken by the view of the sun rising over the mountains. Every morning was like the first morning of creation, he said. He described these dawn epiphanies as if he was the luckiest man alive. And I think in some ways he believed himself to be just that.

Ben fought for life. When I was with him I felt the power of the life force in his thirst for it. Despite every medical prediction, he survived to attend his niece's wedding.

The following day he left a long message on my answering machine describing the celebration. Yes, he considered himself the most fortunate man alive. I saved that message for a long time. I wanted to keep it forever, but somewhere along the line it was deleted.

He fought for me as well. Although I was in the midst of my reprieve and he was fading before my eyes, he worried about me and prayed for me and wanted to protect me. When I told him that Nurse Ratchet from Day Oncology had ripped the drip from the back of my hand instead of easing it out gently at the end of the session, he was outraged. That afternoon, as he was being wheeled downstairs from his room for a CT scan, he insisted on detouring to Day Oncology, where he lodged a complaint on my behalf.

Ben was having that particular scan because he was scheduled for an operation that would most likely kill him. He wasn't strong enough for such serious surgery, but there seemed to be no alternative. A huge tumor was blocking his intestines, and without the operation he was sure to die.

Ben later told me that as he was being fed into the scanner he had a vision of me, my body, totally cancer-free. He insisted that it wasn't a fantasy. It was a simple truth. I believed him. I still believe him.

The scan showed that Ben's tumor had mysteriously shifted and was no longer blocking any vital organs. No one could explain it. His doctors were astounded. Ben was released from hospital. He lived for another three months, against anyone's wildest expectations, and he greeted each day as the gift that it was.

To me, Ben was a man who had been awakened to the path of right living. In the final weeks of his life he radiated a goodness, a holiness that I had never before encountered. He seemed to have a foot in both worlds, like a bridge.

When he was too weak to remain at home with his friends and his garden and his marijuana cookies, he moved to a hospice "just to learn a bit more about pain management," he assured me. Doug and I visited him often during the week that he was there. I was upset that his room looked out on a brick wall. Where was the view he'd had at St. Katherine's? Where were his dawn epiphanies? Ben didn't mind. He smiled and I saw from the light in his eyes that he had all the dawn and all the epiphanies he needed.

The question I wanted to ask was: would I be as calm and as radiant when my time came? Would I in fact be here, in this very hospice, in the not-too-distant future? Every time I walked into the place, my soul trembled.

There was no flesh left on Ben's body. He was literally a skeleton draped in skin, yet when we came to see him, he got up, he put on his dressing gown, and sat with us. Until he couldn't. The last time I saw him conscious, he hugged me, and despite his skeletal state, I felt that of the two of us he was the stronger, that he was still protecting me.

He hugged me, and I hugged him back, this body that no longer shielded my sight from the pure spirit within.

"That's my soul to your soul." The last words I heard him say.

My connection with Ben does not end there. Since his first bout with pancreatic cancer six years earlier, Ben had been writing his memoirs. Some months before he died, when I was visiting him in hospital, he hesitantly asked if I would edit them. Ben was much more adept at giving than he was at taking, so I welcomed the opportunity to do something for him. The editing didn't take long. It wasn't a long manuscript, and apart from correcting spelling and grammar and rearranging sentences to clarify their meaning, I left it as it was.

Ben wrote the way he spoke, with the same colloquialisms, the same straightforward diction, the same warm-hearted, sometimes heated enthusiasm. I was drawn to his book, for all its quirkiness. He told his story simply, without literary adornments. The edited version remained with him. I knew that he was proud of having accomplished this, but I didn't know how I could help him to take it further. Finally, when he moved to the hospice, it hit me. You don't need a publisher to make a book, not even a vanity publisher. All you need is a copy of the manuscript, which I had, and an outlet of Quick Printing, which was at the end of my street.

Doug and I took the manuscript to Quick Printing, chose a vinyl cover, good-quality paper and binding, and ordered thirty-six copies. Thirty-six is an auspicious number in Jewish tradition, and in his latter years, Ben, like Doug and I, put great store in Jewish tradition. Adam and Eve inhabited the Garden of Eden for thirty-six hours before being exiled. At Hanukkah, the "festival of lights," we light thirty-six candles over an eight-day period. There are thirty-six volumes of the Talmud, the "oral law" known as the "hidden light of Torah." And throughout history, the life of the world is said to have depended upon thirty-six "hidden *tzaddikim*," righteous people who secretly sustain the world, without receiving credit for their work. I believe that Ben was one of those hidden lights, whose spirit sustains all life.

We told the manager of Quick Printing about Ben, and he promised to fill the order as soon as possible. Still, it took a day and a half. As soon as they were ready, we rushed the copies to the hospice. Ben was sleeping, deeply, so Doug left the books beside his bed.

Ben died the following day, but in the interim he woke, found the books, and managed to give signed copies to his mother, his sisters, his nieces and nephews. Afterwards, his sister tried to describe to me how much joy the book brought him. She didn't have to. As a writer myself, I understood. After Ben's death, his family had more copies made to give to family and friends. Ben's book was quoted by the rabbi at his funeral, and at the consecration of his tombstone, and at a memorial service held a year after his death. At all these gatherings I overheard people talking about the book, about how much insight it gave them into Ben, about how their reading it drew them closer to him even after his death. I don't think I have ever been as proud of an act as I am of this.

Perhaps it's the joy I brought him in his final hours, or its imprint, that has kept Ben so firmly and unquestionably in my life. No one has ever remained so close to me after their death.

Certain moments with Ben, when he handed me his manuscript, when he insisted on carrying a chair for me, when he told me of his vision beneath the CT scanner, remain imprinted within me. But the actual stamp, the encounter that makes all the other imprints, is the last time I saw him conscious, when he hugged me and said, "That's my soul to your soul."

It was one of those moments that don't really belong in this world. Ben was by then not entirely here. He had one foot in another world. He was as emaciated as anyone I've ever seen, live or in a photograph, but his voice was strong, as if it came from elsewhere. "My soul to your soul." I know it sounds strange, some might say crazy, but I didn't hear him in the way one usually hears a communication from one person to another. It wasn't "language" that by its very nature loses its essence in the act of articulation. It was a transmission. "My soul to your soul." No barriers. Nothing was lost in translation. Perhaps he never said it. Well, I know that he did because Doug heard him as well. What I'm trying to say – and as I try I am again reminded of how clumsy language can be – is that he didn't need to say it. It would still have been said.

I have never been partial to tales of apparitions and the other world, but I cannot understand this any other way. Something of Ben entered my soul and lodged there. I sense his presence as frequently now as I did right after his death, one and a half years ago. Perhaps my own neediness has created a fantasy, a recipe for salvation, but reasonable as that explanation may be, I don't buy it. Ben has convinced me that there is some enduring presence after death.

I know how strange it sounds, but I believe that somehow, he does watch over me. Not long after his funeral, in the midst of a bout of severe "scanxiety," fearing that I would soon be following him, I heard by chance an old song by Bob Dylan.

Soul to soul,
Our shadows roll,
And I'll be with you when the deal goes down.

I can't help it. I really believe that he will be with me, and crazy or not, my faith in that has largely conquered my fear, my indescribable horror of death.

17

Bella and I first met across a desk, so to speak. She was a student in one of my adult Jewish education classes. I can't remember which one. Something mystical. "A Mystical Reading of the Book of Genesis," "Mystical Exodus," "Introduction to Kabbalah," "A Mystic's Guide to Festivals and Fast Days." That's all I really knew how to teach. I compiled courses of eight two-hour sessions, and the school employed me to teach them one evening per week.

I barely remember Bella from those classes. She was very quiet. The only reason I remember her at all, I think, is because of her striking looks. She was a tall woman, dark, statuesque, with high cheekbones and a careworn face. A little smile often played upon her lips. She had a marked South African accent.

Bella and I became friends when she started coming to the classes I taught from my home. Before I became ill, I taught from home on Wednesday evenings as well as Thursday mornings. During the day, Bella worked as a pharmacist, so she came to the evening class. Sometimes she stayed after class and we chatted. There was a kind of gentle nobility about her. Perhaps she was born that way, or perhaps she was shaped by her experiences. At any rate, when I heard her story I came to appreciate the lines carved into her forehead and around her eyes. Bella had two daughters and a son. In their early twenties, both daughters had been struck by cancer. One had fully recovered, and the other had also survived, but with damaged kidneys. She was on dialysis, awaiting a transplant. Bella shared her story one evening after another woman, who'd also stayed back to talk, told us of a son with developmental problems. I'd also pitched in with my own maternal distress, regarding a child who had gone off the rails. Opening our hearts to each other like that inevitably forged a bond between us. We were all in pain over our children, but when Bella spoke about her daughters, I was struck dumb. Before my illness, the very word "cancer" tended to paralyze me. Two daughters! How had she borne it? I suspected that this explained her air of nobility as well as her careworn face.

After that evening, I considered Bella a friend. We didn't see each other socially, but we talked often after class. I admired her. She was softly spoken, a gentle woman, yet strong. Tall and strong. Looking back, I wonder if I avoided a more intimate relationship because of my fear of cancer. Before I got it myself, I managed to remain remarkably disentangled from those who had been touched by it.

After my initial diagnosis I dropped the Wednesday evening classes. Bella sent me a few emails. She may have called once or twice. I was too shell-shocked to take anything in. Some months later, when I was settling into my post-chemo reprieve, she reappeared in my life. A friend of mine, an ultra-Orthodox woman, had organized a circle of women to recite psalms and to pray for those in need of healing. I was on the prayer list that she updated and sent out by email each month, and although I knew that others were praying for me, I wasn't fulfilling my duty to pray for others. I felt guilty about this, but not yet guilty enough to do anything about it. That would come later.

In Jewish tradition, the prayer for the sick cites the Hebrew name of the person in need and the Hebrew name of his or her mother. Not knowing people's Hebrew names, I hardly ever recognized any names on the list. One day, however, when I was glancing at the most recent prayer list, I saw the name "Bella," followed by an appeal for someone to send in her Hebrew name and the Hebrew name of her mother. Something twisted in the pit of my stomach, as it had when I'd first received that call from the breast-screen clinic. I didn't know how I knew, but I knew.

Bella called me later that evening.

"Yes," she said. "It's me. I've got lung cancer."

Bella had never smoked a cigarette in her life. Aside from her two daughters, there was no cancer that she knew of in her family. How could this be? She wondered if she and her daughters had been exposed to some kind of radiation when they were living in South Africa.

Bella had an operation that left her weak and debilitated. When she was well enough, she had a course of radiotherapy. I visited her in hospital after the operation, and later she'd visit me at home on her way back from radiotherapy. We'd take walks together. She was still the tall, gentle woman I'd got to know in those after-class chats. Unable to continue working, she began to reflect upon her life. The more she revealed of herself, the more I saw that her strength was always for others. She gave unstintingly, unconditionally, to her children, to her husband, to her elderly mother, to her friends. Her surgeon told her that he had most likely removed the cancer with the operation, and if there were any stray cells remaining, the radiotherapy would mop them up. She felt confident that she would overcome this, just as her daughters had overcome their cancers. But like many of us who are facing life-threatening illness, the illness gave her pause, and she tried to take stock of her life. She was an outstanding daughter, wife, and mother, but she wanted to find a passion, a creative outlet outside of her family obligations. Looking back, I think she found it in the passion of her search, inside her passionate longing for something to give meaning to her life.

On her birthday, when we were both enjoying a reprieve from our cancers, I joined Bella for a walk on the beach. For a while we walked sedately along the paved seaside track, but when we reached the end, we took off our shoes and ran onto the sand and danced, and danced. Bella had lung cancer. I had breast cancer. I was in my early fifties. She was in her late fifties. Our worlds had capsized, our future was bleak, and we danced, and we laughed. Bella was a strong woman, a passionate woman. I often wish that she had known how strong, how passionate she was.

As the months went by, and the dates for our respective scans approached, we comforted and supported each other. Bella's scan was supposed to tell her that her lung cancer had disappeared. It didn't. She did a long round of heavy-duty chemo. It didn't help. She tried more radiation. The cancer kept growing. She sought second and third opinions. No one could offer her any help, or any hope. My chemo reprieve had also ended suddenly and cruelly. We spoke regularly on the phone, sometimes for hours, reflecting, bewailing, weeping, and laughing.

Bella remained her tall, strong, and gentle self, even as her physical strength waned. She began to have difficulty breathing. Her lungs were filling with fluid, so once a week she went to the hospital to have them drained. At home, she needed an oxygen mask a lot of the time. After a while, she stopped trying to climb up and down the stairs every day and remained in bed. She was visited daily by a hospice nurse, yet as far as I could see, Bella remained the bulwark of her family. Not long before she died, her daughter received her long-awaited kidney transplant. Bella lived to see the transplant take, and her daughter begin to recover. Bella was so very strong, and she never stopped giving of her strength. When she died, her family was set adrift, so Bella gave them something strong enough to pull them back together, something strong enough to hold them together.

Ben was one of the last of our community to be buried at the old Jewish cemetery, before it was declared full. Bella was one of the first to be buried at the new Jewish cemetery, which is much further away from the center of Melbourne. The new cemetery is in the middle of nowhere, surrounded by open fields. The day of Bella's funeral was wet. The cemetery grounds were muddy. The crowd was so large that many of us had to wait outside the chapel and listen in the rain. By the time the mourners gathered to follow the funeral procession to the gravesite, Doug and I were drenched. The rain had cleared, but it was bitterly cold.

Traditionally, the congregation remains silent while the rabbi recites the graveside prayers, and the principal mourners recite the Kaddish, but as Bella was lowered into her open grave, people began to point and to gasp. They couldn't help themselves. The most perfect, most gigantic rainbow I have ever seen suddenly filled the sky, a huge multi-hued arch peaking exactly above Bella's grave. The bleak, forbidding landscape was transformed into an orchard of love. Thankfully, one of the mourners had enough presence of mind and disrespect of convention to covertly take a picture. But as I saw the faces of Bella's children reflect the glow of the rainbow, I doubted that they would ever need a photograph to remind them of this moment.

Bella was a very strong woman.

The deaths of Ben and Bella, and of others since, leave me feeling as if I live my life on a battlefield, that I fight on with the bodies of the slain strewn around me.

Lately, life with cancer has also seemed like a boxing match. I use my reprieves to swallow life in huge gulps, I squeeze cool fresh water over my overheated brow, and when the reprieve ends I stagger back into the ring, to take more of whatever medicine is being dished up this time around.

During that year of my first reprieve, when I loved and lost Ben and Bella, I hovered between bouts of terror and moments of revelation and exhilaration. I didn't swing between them. That was the problem. I was pulled between them. Some parts of me – my feet – were buried in the earth, unable to free themselves from the awful medical truth that I was not going to live much longer, while at the same time my head was up in the clouds, floating in the certainty of future health. The problem was that these two parts of me couldn't communicate. I desperately wanted the certainty of that part of me that was up in the clouds to transmit its wisdom to the part that had one foot in the grave, but I couldn't. At times I feared that I may go mad.

18

It was during this period that I reconnected with Doris, the psychologist. I'd seen her once before, a week after I'd received the awful results of the lung biopsy. I'd just had the stitches from the biopsy removed. I was still in a lot of pain and a great deal of shock, and I wanted a miracle, now.

Doug dropped me off at Doris's and arranged to be waiting outside an hour later when our session was due to end.

Doris was kind and sympathetic. She told me her own cancer story. She explained why I should not rely on statistics, and gave very convincing reasons.

"Statistics can only describe and predict outcomes for a group of people. They can't accurately predict what will happen to an individual within the group. An individual's path and outcome may be very different from that taken by the group as a whole." It made sense. Her voice was lyrical and reassuring.

She explained hypnotherapy and told me of her own experience with it. But I was in pain and my head was spinning. She kept me there way past the hour. I felt trapped. I was a child again, unable to state my needs, yearning for my bed, my pillow, worrying about Doug waiting out in the car. And Doris wasn't handing me a miracle cure. No "get out of jail free" card. She was just talking, and I sat opposite her, mute.

I knew of and greatly admired Doris as a poet. I knew she was a highly qualified psychologist who specialized in treating cancer patients. I'd heard of her genius for hypnotherapy. I suppose I expected her to be superhuman, to simply know what was going on inside me when she'd never met me before, and I wasn't giving her the slightest clue. Why was I unable to simply state my needs? I suspect it was because I was so desperate to hand her my power. She was an amazing woman. She would do a much better job with the mess that was me than I ever could.

After close to two hours, I was released. Doug had waited patiently outside because he thought I was getting something I needed. I fell into the passenger seat and burst into tears. I was totally overwhelmed.

"I'm never going back!"

"Okay," said Doug.

I called her the next day and explained that I didn't feel ready for hypnotherapy.

"That's fine," she said. Her voice was so kind, so reassuring, so non-judgmental. I was flooded with a desire to see her again, but I resisted.

"Call me when you think you're ready," she said.

I hung up, feeling both relief and grief.

I went to a teacher of meditation instead. Nan had been recommended by a mutual friend who described her as "old and wise." That was all I needed to hear.

Doug dropped me at her beautiful Victorian home in Brighton, near the beach. Her garden was magnificent and well loved. When she opened the door and led me through the formal dining room into the living area, I was transported back to my childhood, but whereas my visit to Doris had sent me spinning into the sad childhood, now I was taken to the happy one. The polished wood, the portraits on the wall, the wonderful, comforting smell of wood and flowers and wisdom. I was in my grandmother's home! When Nan began to speak in that broad and slightly croaky Australian accent, just like my grandmother, I wanted to fall into her arms. I shed forty years, and I was comforted.

"Why have you come to see me?" she asked.

I'd given her the bare bones of my story over the phone, so I realized that she wasn't asking directly about the cancer.

"Well," I said, "when I heard about you I just knew I had to come. If I want to live to be an old and wise woman, I need to learn from one."

"Harrumph!" she grumbled. "Called me old, did he? I'll give him old! I'm not old,

I'm mature." The last two words were uttered in a nasal, upper-class accent.

I smiled. She harrumphed again.

And then we meditated. I sat on her well-stuffed grandmotherly couch, and she sat opposite in her favorite armchair. Flowering tendrils tapped on the window and birds twittered from the trees. Now and then we heard the sound of a train passing and beyond that, the ocean. It was a cold day. An electric wall heater warmed the room.

On Nan's instruction, I removed my shoes, placed my feet side by side on the floor, and rested my hands palm-down on my knees. I closed my eyes and breathed gently, in and out, through my nose.

After a while, she began to talk.

"Be still," she said. "Right now, there is nothing you need to be doing. This is your time for healing."

Be still? Nothing I needed to do? How could I not have known how much I'd longed to hear those words? In an instant, I realized what I'd denied myself for years, for decades. I'd denied myself my self. A floodgate lifted and my eyes leaked tears. I sat there with my stockinged feet on the floor, my hands on my knees, and the tears leaked from my closed eyes. It was wonderful.

Nan gave me tapes and I listened to them at home, every day, all alone, in my own private space, in my own private time. This was the time when there was absolutely nothing for me to do but to sit and be still. I didn't even have to worry.

My visits to Nan and her meditation tapes helped me through those first eight weeks of chemo, and on into my period of reprieve. I learned to tune in to the silence within. It wasn't just a cliché after all. It actually worked. Once in a while, quite rarely, I had a small epiphany.

And that's how I reconnected with Doris. A few months into my reprieve, I achieved one of those rare moments of real meditation. I actually entered that part of me, the core that always knows exactly what to do. And I knew it was time to call Doris.

She agreed to see me the following week, which was incredibly gracious. I knew that she hardly ever took new patients and was booked up months in advance. Was she giving me a second chance, or did she consider that first strange encounter all those months ago as part of something that was still unfolding?

This time we connected beautifully. Our common love of language, and especially of imagery, bonded us almost immediately. I told Doris of my fears and she translated them into wonderful, redemptive scenarios. She has a beautiful mind.

Predictably, I was an ideal subject for hypnotherapy. I've always had a good imagination, and when someone speaks as beautifully as Doris, concocting such marvelous imaginary worlds, I will enter willingly. Most of our sessions were spent talking, but often, just before the end, Doris would suggest a little hypnotherapy and I would willingly acquiesce. I'd draw up the footrest and lie back in the recliner chair, closing my eyes with a little trick she taught me that never failed to induce deep relaxation almost instantly, and Doris would talk.

The hypnotic state, if that is what I was in, is not what I would have once imagined. I was very relaxed. Doris's voice often seemed to come from inside my own head, but as far as I know I never lost consciousness. I'm sure that if I'd had to, I could have woken myself up at any time. I never tried. I loved the worlds she took me into, and often, when she declared the end and "counted me awake," I emerged reluctantly, wishing I could remain inside the story a little longer.

Under hypnosis, Doris helped me connect my head in the clouds with my feet in the earth by gently reminding me of the process of photosynthesis. The hard facts on the ground did not have to be severed from the heavenly promises of miraculous redemption. Instead they could be nourished and transformed by them.

I came away from Doris with images of ballerinas dancing in absolute stillness, of oily puddles on the road turning to rainbows in unexpected sunlight, of houses filled with unexplored rooms, of new worlds filled with possibility.

Some of these sessions she taped for me to take home and listen to again. I collected four or five such tapes and listened to them repeatedly during those months of my first reprieve. It took a while, quite a long while, but finally I got it. All the stories, all the beautiful images, were telling me the same thing. In varied but equally stunning ways, just one single message was being planted in my subconscious. By the time it popped into my conscious mind, it had already taken hold, and my days were already guided by it. It was the message I needed most, the one without which my life with cancer would have no color, no quality, no joy.

With her stories, Doris was telling me, or my subconscious, over and over, in a myriad of ways, that there was nothing for her to tell me because I already knew. I, and no one else. My path, my guiding light, was already written within me, and nowhere else. I had been looking for a savior, for someone to pull me out from under the car, to carry me up from the bottom of the pool. But I already had all the help I needed. The more I internalized this fact, the less I worried over the endless stream of advice I was receiving on everything from my diet to my spiritual blemishes. The answer was within me. Finally, I was empowered.

With this in mind, it's not surprising that the most powerful image of all was one I received from myself, not from Doris. I had been sitting in my "meditation chair," listening to one of her tapes. I must have nodded off. I remember feeling overcome by drowsiness. I remember Doris's voice trailing off. I guess I had a dream, but it seemed more like a vision. I walked into a bare, cell-like room, not like a prisoner's cell, more like a monk's. An elderly Jew was sitting stooped over a workbench, facing a small window. I don't recall seeing anything through the window. The man's gabardined back was facing the door, so when I entered I couldn't see what he was doing. A large, black, velvet skullcap covered most of his relatively large head, and wisps of silvery hair lay on his long neck. His build was slim and wiry. When he shifted his position and sighed, I saw one long, curled sidelock spring away from his cheek. I ventured further into the room and saw his hands, his long, elegant, nimble fingers, his beard almost touching the workbench, which was strewn with bits and pieces of clocks: wheels and pins and screws, and fragile hour, minute, and second hands. He was putting together a very delicate watch, my silver watch. It was a beautiful sight. Then he spoke, gently, firmly, enthusiastically, in a voice I could only describe as timeless.

"I know it's been fixed before, but this time I'm fixing it forever." A finger came up and wound itself around a sidelock.

I never saw his face. I awoke, or came to, with a start, brimming with joy and relief. I was going to be okay!

I told Doris of my dream-vision at our next session. She was visibly excited. I could see she considered this a very positive development. Perhaps she saw more than she admitted to and was waiting for me to discover it for myself, or perhaps I really was the only one holding the key, but it was weeks before I finally realized the deeper meaning of the dream.

I was in the shower, pressing away at my left breast, checking on the existing lump and probing for others. I performed these in-shower breast exams frequently, probably obsessively. When I did them I pictured my breast the way oncologists and radiologists saw it, with the nipple in the center and the breast itself divided into three-dimensional slices, like a cake, or a clock. Medical people used the clock analogy. My initial diagnoses had included two major breast lesions, one at five o'clock and one at one o'clock. The one at five o'clock had disappeared after that first round of chemo. In the shower, I moved my fingers to five o'clock. Nothing but soft, beautiful breast flesh. Then I probed around one o'clock. The lump was still there, but it didn't feel any bigger. I let the hot water wash away the soap, my mind moving lazily. Then it hit me, not like a thunderbolt or a lightning strike. More like something I'd always known, but had been too slow minded to realize. The watchmaker was referring to the source of my cancer! He was fixing me, healing me, permanently.

I rushed out of the shower and assaulted Doug with my discovery. He was impressed. Doug believes that the key to any individual's story can be found in the annals of that person's family. He is an experienced genealogist, so it didn't take him long to discover a link with my not-too-distant past. My great-great-grandfather, Joseph Masel, had been a jeweler and watchmaker.

I couldn't wait to tell Doris that I'd solved the riddle. When I breathlessly related the whole story at our next session, she beamed.

19

My father's great-grandfather was the professional watchmaker in the family, but my mother's father was the fixer who lives on in my memory. He loved collecting bits and pieces and putting them back together. He'd walk for hours around Sydney, a small man with well-oiled, thick, silver hair and a mouthful of gold teeth, collecting broken radios, discarded bits of machinery, and especially broken clocks and watches. He would arrive home with the jacket pockets of his worn, grey Jewish Polish immigrant's suit bulging with booty. He'd stash the stuff in a large room under his house. "Unda needa da hoss," he called it, with his Yiddish inflection, and so did the grandchildren. The place was a kid's delight, a treasure trove, like my grandfather's teeth. He'd sit at his long wooden workbench, humming bits of songs he remembered from his childhood, putting the watches and clocks back together, often replacing broken parts with pieces from earlier finds. The finished products he gave to us.

"What for?" my grandmother would shout from upstairs. "*Fa vuss*? Stop the *meshugas* and let the little ones get out into the sunshine!"

I never tired of looking at the delicate mechanics of a watch when my grandfather had taken the back off it and exposed it in all its glory. It was like a human body, each part with its own special function, its own working relationship with the other parts, all moving in harmony, like a vast melodious universe.

My grandfather was not a practical man. He never adjusted to life in Australia. He and my grandmother had arrived from Poland with nothing. She began by selling flowers at Paddy's Market in Sydney, but she soon became a successful businesswoman. Back in the 1940s, Australia was as remote from Europe as we are today from the moon, and the upper classes couldn't tell a French accent from a Polish one. Calling herself "Madame Koupier," my grandmother supported the family by decorating the homes of wealthy Anglo-Saxon families in the latest "French décor" while my grandfather Avraham Koopershmit from Bialystok collected flotsam and jetsam, bits and pieces of other people's lives, and put them back together. He also put together stories – wonderful stories of snowy forest adventures, and children who accomplished great things, and witches and fairies who prepared great feasts and sang like birds.

My grandfather often came to see us in Melbourne from his home in Sydney and stayed a while. At bedtime, he would hang his suit jacket, shiny with age, on a hook above my open window. I think he only had that one old-fashioned pre-war Polish suit. It had a special smell, not obnoxious, not to me anyway. It was the smell of well-oiled, ticking watches and melodious universes. My grandfather washed regularly, but he didn't believe in soap or shampoo, because they destroyed "the natural oils." He lived well into his nineties, but went a little loopy before the end. Living in a small flat, without his practical wife to constrain him, the piles of bits and pieces grew around him until there was no room to sort and to fix, no room to move. He sat amongst the rubble and ate birdseed until my mother persuaded him to move to an aged-care center, where, bereft of his beloved chaos, he died after a few months.

He had separated from my grandmother while I was still a child. Their lifestyles were completely incompatible. My grandmother loved light and modern kitchens and card parties and panoramic views of Sydney Harbour. My grandfather wanted to sit in silence in the gloom and fix his bits and pieces. Burning too many lights after dark was just a waste of money, he said, or rather shouted. Some said he was miserly, but I believed he just didn't need that much light in order to see. He saw in a different way. Despite the separation, he and my grandmother never really parted. Twice a day, every day of the year, he would walk for twenty minutes from his apartment to hers, every day, year in year out, for lunch and dinner, gefilte fish, matzo balls, chopped liver, schnitzel, sweet carrots, red cabbage with sultanas, which she would serve as befits a decent wife, watching over his nutrition, and criticizing his lifestyle.

And when he came with her to Melbourne and visited us at night, he hung up his old suit jacket, the pockets jingling with the bits and pieces he'd picked up along the way, and waited for the wind to enter the window and fill the jacket with life, and make it dance. Then the story could begin.

Perhaps my childhood was not so extraordinarily sad after all. When I remember my grandfather's stories and the soft belly of our black cocker spaniel and the early-morning rides in the horse-driven cart that delivered milk to all the houses on our street, I can see that perhaps, like most people, I had two childhoods. In the happy childhood one happy memory triggers another, and on and on they go, gently bobbing waves in a clear blue sea. In the unhappy childhood, the same process occurs. One memory triggers another, and before I know it I'm trapped inside, looking for a sliver of light.

Could my happiness or otherwise today possibly depend upon which childhood I choose to inhabit? Would dwelling in the happy memories make this cancer easier to bear?

My life with cancer has already clocked up its own good times and its bad times, although it's nowhere distant enough, and perhaps even with distance it is simply not possible to differentiate, as I can so easily with my childhood. My friend and teacher Avivah Zornberg once mentioned the word "dappled" in this context, and it has stayed with me. Today, I looked out of my bedroom window and saw the light of the sun dappled by the leaves of the great oak tree; a dappled light dancing on its huge trunk. That is life. That could be life. That would be a meaningful life.

The months of my first reprieve were dappled. Ben died a horrible but beautiful and saintly death. Bella faded like a great oak tree brittle and withered by drought, but she was a strong woman. She brought us blessed rain, and a rainbow that filled our sky. The story of Bella's rainbow will surely be passed down through the generations in her family, like the story of the exodus from Egypt.

And in those months Doris helped me find a path, more of a nebulous track, through the aftermath of an advanced cancer diagnosis.

The pathway I discovered with Doris's help was one I'd actually physically traversed early in my first reprieve. Still reeling from the effects of the chemo, I'd agreed to travel north to a luxury health retreat with my longtime friend Dena. The retreat featured gourmet organic cuisine, yoga, Tai Chi, five-star accommodation, lots of yin, heaps of yang, and for a phenomenal extra cost added to the already phenomenal daily rate, one of the most luxurious and multifarious spas in the country.

It was an utter extravagance and we were determined to have fun. The retreat was hidden in the mostly unpopulated hills behind Queensland's popular Gold Coast. The place was stunning, with sweeping views all the way out to the Pacific Ocean and, closer to hand, rainforest and bushland ringing with wildlife. It was built like a tiny village, with renovated heritage houses transported piece by piece from their original locations. The retreat was five-star eco-chic. We loved it. The food was unbelievable and very artistically presented, for which I was grateful, as I had not yet regained my appetite and mostly enjoyed its aesthetic qualities.

Dena and I had booked for three days, but by the third day, as is our wont, we rebelled. We forwent the dawn Tai Chi on the hill with the beautiful vista, and the early-morning bushwalk, and the meditation session and the Pilates. Enough! It was time to abandon bodymindandsoul. I was too tired and she was too bored. It was a cold and drizzly morning. After breakfast (which we did not abandon) I decided to spend a few hours resting in our lavish ranch-style apartment. She said she'd go for a walk.

As I left the dining room intending to return to our suite, the rain abated and a weak sun appeared. I decided to seize the moment and take a short solitary walk. Since my diagnosis, I had been watched over so well and so carefully that I had seldom been alone. I headed for the other side of the property, where I'd been told there were horses and chickens in a coop, and a vegetable garden. It didn't take long to find them. I was alone on the farm with the chicks and the forest sounds and the wet vegetables and the muddy path. After all the retreat activities of the past few days, it was good to taste a morsel of real solitude. A degree of sadness lifted from me. I felt a little lighter. The rain returned, but softly, and I enjoyed its gentle falling.

I started back, trudging in the mud, intending to spend the rest of the morning quietly, with a book. On the way I just had to stop on the hill where we met for early-morning Tai Chi. I could see through the dark wet morning to the choppy sea. No one was about, so I stood tall in the rain and tried to remember the Tai Chi moves I'd practiced with the aid of a DVD at home in Melbourne. I must have looked like a clumsy oversized wet emu, but I felt graceful. I raised my arms in silent salute, and let go of another degree of sadness.

I didn't see Dena approach until she called out to me. She was with John, the resident gardener, who we'd heard was no ordinary gardener, but a recipient of the Order of the British Empire for his services to horticulture and, by the look of him, all things green. He was a good-looking, leathery man, rustic, fair-haired, bearded with sturdy boots, knowing blue eyes, and a sensitive, weather-lined face, like a poet's. It was the face of someone who had suffered and survived.

John had offered to take Dena on a hike. They invited me along. I hesitated. It was wet, my canvas shoes were already drenched, I had no raincoat, and I was tired, chemo tired.

"We'll go slow," said John. "We won't leave you behind."

An old spirit for adventure stirred in me. The day had become colder. The rain was now biting. Dena's eyes sparkled like they had years ago when she and I decided on the spur of the moment to drive 7,000 kilometers with young kids and no husbands to the center of Australia and back. How could I refuse now? It wasn't another trip to the outback, but I was breaking loose, just a little.

We left the established path and started making our way through the dripping trees down a sharp decline. The ground was slippery. I trod carefully and every now and then John reached out his hand and helped me down. The place was magical. Dappled light, everywhere. This was a special descent. It already had an air of mystery. John identified various trees and plants and briefly outlined the long history of the land, but mostly we were silent, listening to the sounds of the forest. Birdsong, now and then a kookaburra laugh, and the rustling of land-bound creatures of the bush. This was a heartland, a place of wealth, where sadness was permitted and tears could not be told from rain.

Dena and I heard the gurgling of rushing water together. A little further down the slope we saw the stream, more of a river after the overnight rain, beautiful and fast, and on the other side, a sharp incline.

"Okay, ladies," said John. "This is where we cross."

What had I gotten myself into? I was weaker than I'd been since childhood, exhausted, nauseous, tottering on my feet. How could I cross that river?

John held out a hand. "We'll take it stone by stone. Piece of cake."

He went first, with me in the middle and Dena bringing up the rear. The stones were slippery. My shoes were soaked. My immune system was weak. I could be catching pneumonia. I didn't care. I grasped John's hand and struggled, stone by slippery stone, to the other side, where we sat on a jutting rock, laughing, surveying our path through the water.

"Told you," he said. "Piece of cake."

The way back was hard, the incline was steep. We stopped frequently, but I could barely catch my breath. My lungs were bursting. It was madness.

"There's only one way home," said John, "so you're gonna have to keep going."

And then I saw the twinkle in his eye. He was taking two of the luxury resort's middle-aged guests, one with incurable breast cancer, on a dangerous unscheduled hike. He knew exactly what he was doing. John deserved his OBE, and more.

I staggered into the resort, supported by John and Dena, feeling like Rocky after he'd run up all those steps. I wished they'd hold up my limp arms in victory. Something special had happened. I had forged my path.

I paid for the adventure with a nasty cold and a miserable few weeks, but it was worth it.

Yes, I thought, I had it all figured out. The path, the process, the program. Yep, right up until it all collapsed around me. The reprieve had lasted so long, and I was feeling so good, that on some level I had convinced myself that the game was over and I'd won. I'd scored a knockout in the first round. I'd been having my scans every three months. The few remaining lesions were growing ever so slightly, and I had become accustomed to Lara's assurance that all was well for another three months. No need to go back onto chemo. When I called Nuclear Medicine to book a scan for early October, I was a little disconcerted when told that the only available time was the day before Yom Kippur, the Day of Atonement, but my confidence was riding high. I took it for a good sign.

They say that on Yom Kippur, God pulls out His infamous Books of Life and Death, and writes each of us into one or the other. I was to have my scans the day before Yom Kippur and get the results the day after. On Yom Kippur 5769, 2008 in the Gregorian calendar, my life would literally hang in the balance, as I inhabited that dreaded limbo time when my future was sealed, but I did not yet know it.

That year, on the eve of Yom Kippur, at the Kol Nidrei service, I was to deliver the sermon to our assembled community.

I'd taken on this task the year before as well. Giving the *drasha* on the eve of Yom Kippur had quickly become a sort of sacred rite, a commitment to life. Not long after the lung metastases were first diagnosed, Mark, the president of our congregation had sent me a curt email.

"You're giving the Kol Nidrei *drasha*."

A *drasha* is not really a sermon, not to me, anyway. I think of it as a discourse, at its best an intimate talk, an outpouring of the soul, a journey into the depth of Torah text, into the place where its truth touches our own.

As far as *drasha*s go, the Kol Nidrei service on the eve of Yom Kippur is an annual highlight. Our community attracts between four and five hundred worshipers for Kol Nidrei, many of whom rarely open a prayer book or think of going to synagogue during the rest of the year. But on Kol Nidrei, there's barely a Jew who will not show up at some synagogue, somewhere. On the eve of Yom Kippur, as on the eve of Passover, Jews who generally have neither time nor patience for ancient ritual remember that they are Jews.

Our community is named Shira Hadasha, meaning "new song." It seeks to promote women's participation and an egalitarian approach from within an Orthodox framework. We want the rituals that link us all the way back to the ancients, and we each want a voice. It works for me. Mark was an old friend, and shaken to the core by the news of my illness. I sensed the single-mindedness in his curt email.

"You're giving the Kol Nidrei *drasha*."

"What if I'm not well enough?" I responded. *What if I'm dead?* I thought. "I'll need backup."

"No backup. You're doing it."

Mark is responsible for our community. If I didn't show, hundreds of people would be left without words of spiritual uplift on the holiest night of the year.

"No backup." The oncologist at Worthington Hospital had told my mother that he doubted I'd last the year.

"No backup." Mark's short reply was up there with the greatest expressions of faith I'd ever heard.

And so the Kol Nidrei *drasha* became my annual commitment to life.

The first year, I told a tale from the treasure house of the great Hassidic storyteller, Rebbe Nachman of Bratzlav. Well, what I actually told was a story within a story within a story within "The Story of the Seven Beggars." That's part of Rebbe Nachman's genius; his stories truly imitate life.

The story I told was about a mountain spring of pure water. This spring existed beyond the world, beyond time. Far away from the mountain spring, deep inside time, was the heart of the world. The heart yearned for the spring, it burned for it, but whenever it tried to traverse the distance between them, it lost its way, because the closer it came to the mountain upon which the spring dwelt, the more perspective it lost, and the less it could see of it. The yearning, burning heart of the world was doomed to remain far from the object of its desire, the spring of pure water.

At the close of each day, when darkness approached, the heart would sing farewell to the spring, and when the spring heard the heart's sad song, it would respond with a beautiful melody of its own. The dying of each day was filled with the call of the broken heart and the response of the spring of pure water; their music filled the world, and thus another day was born.

Rebbe Nachman called each day a new song, born of the death of the previous day. Each day has its own unique melody. The cry of the broken heart, he said, is the source of the greatest blessing of all: the gift of a brand-new day.

The tales of Rebbe Nachman are a world unto themselves. They must be entered into. They require active listening, because no two people can ever experience them in exactly the same way. In that first year of my cancer, the world was born anew for me. I was a wide-eyed child who knew nothing. I no longer had the answer. I barely understood the question. The tales of Rebbe Nachman resist deconstruction. They exist beyond interpretation. This was my Yom Kippur offering.

The following year, on the Yom Kippur that turned out to be the day before the end of my first reprieve, I'd allowed a gloss to cover my sense of mystery. I'd convinced myself into thinking that I might know something, after all. What did I know? After a year and a half of cancer I knew, as I never had before, that life was fragile, that it could end at any moment, that there were no guarantees. As I lived from scan to scan, I'd convinced myself that life was a balancing act, and my task, as if I had any say in it, was to keep from falling.

And so, through my mentor Avivah Zornberg, I came across the funambulist Philippe Petit. In one of her emails, Avivah praised a documentary she'd seen in the States, about a man who had walked a high wire strung between the famous twin towers of the World Trade Center. The film, *Man on Wire*, had not yet been released in Australia. My admiration for Avivah is such that I will follow up on anything she deems worthy of mention. I couldn't wait for the film, so I turned to the Internet, where I read everything I could find on Philippe Petit, the self-described "poet of the high wire" and his famous walk between the twin towers in the summer of 1974. The more I learned the more fascinated I became. Within a few weeks I was obsessed. On the computer I found scraps of the walk that had been filmed, and I watched them over and over. I discovered that Petit had written a book about his "artistic crime of the century," so I trawled the net some more and found a copy with a bookseller in Queensland. I arranged to have it delivered to my home post-haste. I was spending every free minute reading about the walk and watching the film clip over and over. My family noticed my obsession and began to joke about it. Doug developed an antipathy towards the whole thing, especially the hype surrounding it.

But I couldn't let go. Walking the wire, four hundred meters above solid ground. That's what I was doing. That's what we're all doing, whether we know it or not. The thing about Petit was not only that he knew what he was doing, but that he refused to just walk.

He didn't rush across in order to claim the title. He enjoyed himself. He savored the moment. He went back and forth eight times on that August morning in 1974, and he danced. He *danced*, he saluted, he lay on his back with just a wire between life and death and he communed with passing birds. What an image!

The more I read of Philippe Petit, and especially after reading his memoir, the less I liked him personally. He came across as a selfish, ego-driven, uncompassionate "artiste" who was willing to sacrifice everything, including his most devoted friends, at the altar of success. I didn't have much respect for the man, but I couldn't not respect his art. He was a poet. And the image he created on that New York morning skyline, in the midst of the Watergate scandal, was phenomenal.

On the night of Kol Nidrei, in that limbo time between my scans and my results, I stepped off solid ground and out onto the wire, in front of five hundred congregants. No Rebbe Nachman this year. This was not about longing. It was about life and death and the courage to dance one hundred and ten floors above ground level, without a safety net. The thing about Petit, for all his ego-driven behavior, is that he did it. When the time came, he didn't freeze in fear. He didn't stick to the (then) safety of the World Trade Center. And when he stepped out, he didn't stare blindly ahead and race to the other side as quickly as he could, just to prove a point. The guy danced! How could one not be captivated?

The mystics say that when a person steps out onto the thin wire that stretches between twin certainties, between life and death, the prophet Elijah steps out also. And if you listen carefully, they say, you will hear Elijah whispering in your ear. That's how the *Zohar*, the Book of Splendor, came into the world, through the prophet Elijah.

I was told this by a great kabbalist in Jerusalem. He said that if I listened carefully, I would hear the whisper, and if I listened with my inner ear, Elijah would teach me how to tread gently, how to dance upon the wire.

After giving that *drasha*, I felt euphoric. I was walking the wire! I was dancing! But as I was to discover just twenty-four hours later, dancing is fine, until you fall. Then everything falls to pieces.

I spent the entire day of Yom Kippur in synagogue, begging to be written into the Book of Life. I stood by the large picture window that looked out onto the park and watched the sun rise high and then fade as I swayed to the rhythms of the prayers. My *drasha* of the previous evening was still clinging to me, as if I feared a fall. I was in cancer limbo-land, walking the wire, trying to dance. The day was long, and now and then I couldn't help but pick up on the romance of it all.

The final service of Yom Kippur is called Neila, which means "closing." During the day, our concentrated prayers are said to have the power to open all the gates of heaven, giving us a direct line with the Almighty. But the close of the day, when darkness falls, is said to be the holiest time of all. As the gates of heaven close, our words become liquid prayers of desire, slipping through.

The Neila service is always a highlight for me. The approaching end of the twenty-five-hour fast and the hours and hours of prayer surely contribute to my altered, expanded consciousness, but there is also something special about the time itself, inside the fading light, that is uniquely intimate, like an embrace.

Rabbi Hoffman once explained it beautifully. He said that during the Neila service the gates of heaven are closing, but they are not shutting us out. They are closing behind us! In this nowhere twilight time, between twin certainties, all that divides heaven and earth dissolves and nothing stands between us and God.

I always remember his words during the final hours of Yom Kippur. That year, the day before the end of my first reprieve, I felt totally embraced, at one with myself, with God, with destiny.

20

The following afternoon Doug and I were sitting outside Lara's office, waiting for the results of my scans.

I was still high from Yom Kippur and not feeling all that tense. I was getting used to these three-monthly ordeals. Even though we'd had to wait quite a while, Doug and I were chatting calmly when Lara opened her door and invited us in.

She apologized for keeping us waiting.

"No problem," said I, "as long as the news is good."

She didn't respond. As Doug and I settled in the chairs opposite her desk, I saw her face and felt weak.

"Debbie. There are some spots on your brain."

That was enough. I didn't need to hear any more. I'd been in the world of cancer long enough to know that brain metastases would most likely shorten my life-expectancy to a couple of months.

I cried out, a cry from the depths, the cry that is supposed to come on Yom Kippur, and I slumped onto Doug's chest. I squeezed my eyes shut. I didn't want to see. The room was spinning. Doug held me tightly.

"Oh Debbie…" Lara cared. She really cared.

"What do we need to do?" Doug asked.

"There are a few spots there. She'll need an MRI for a clearer picture. Unfortunately, chemo doesn't reach the brain. It can't get past what we call the blood-brain barrier. The options are targeted radiation, or if the spots are too widespread, whole-brain radiation, or possibly surgery. I'm referring her to a radio-oncologist. There's one here at St. Katherine's who I can recommend. I've spoken to her and she's able to fit you in this afternoon."

"Right," said Doug. I was still in hiding, like a kid pulling her sheets up over her head for fear of night monsters.

I moved a little, coming up for air. Lara took a deep breath, as if she was about to go under.

"There's more. The tumors in your lungs have grown considerably. And a couple of those dots, the ones we thought may be scar tissue, have grown. They're not scar tissue. You'll need to go back onto chemo as soon as possible."

I was knocked back down before I'd even regained the floor. I groaned, more of an animal sound than a human one. I grabbed some tissues. My face was streaming. I was not brave. I did not face adversity with fortitude. I did not calmly weigh the options. I certainly did not dance. I freaked. My worst, my darkest, blackest nightmare was being acted out, right now, right here, in Lara's office.

My brain. Not my brain. Please God not my brain.

We had a couple of hours to wait before seeing Karen, the radiation oncologist. Doug and I stumbled out of the hospital and across the road to a small park. I sat on a bench and sobbed. Doug rolled a cigarette and smoked it. He was shaken. He walked as if there was no solid ground beneath his feet. Until that moment I don't think he really believed that I had advanced cancer. He looked to me like a man whose head was in a vise, like he was being forced to face facts. But he pulled himself together. He needed to be there for me. Doug is a precious human being.

Karen, the radio-oncologist, was solicitous, English, and very pretty. She was also forthright, and matter-of-fact.

When we were shown into her office she was looking for the scan that had shown my brain lesions. She had a lot of trouble locating it, and for a few minutes Doug and I allowed ourselves to think that it had all been a terrible mistake, a mix-up, that there were no "spots" on my brain. I smiled, and felt tears of relief rise behind my eyes. When she finally found the scan and showed us the offending spots I had to do another sharp about-face, back toward the darkness.

There were two spots, quite small, on the left side of the cerebellum. She wanted to know if I had trouble with balance, or with my vision. No. I had no symptoms. She thought we'd be able to proceed with targeted radiation, but first I'd need an MRI scan of my brain, for a clearer picture.

The waiting list for MRIs is weeks, sometimes months; but there I was, back at the head of the queue, an urgent case. There are some types of preferential treatment that one hopes never to enjoy. These days, if I have to wait, if no one seems concerned, I feel relieved.

The MRI was booked for the following day. An hour before the appointment, I popped an Ativan to quell my claustrophobia. Perhaps it was the medication, but the scan was not the ordeal I'd imagined it to be. My head was confined inside a tight-fitting cylinder for over half an hour, but I could communicate with the technicians via intercom. I could even see them in their glass booth, as a mirror was strategically positioned just above my eyes. My head was fastened to the bed with a strap and I was forbidden to move it. The scanner made strange, engine-like noises, but I was surprisingly relaxed. I usually panic when I feel trapped. Perhaps being pulled out from under the car all those years ago had given me a faith that I was only now discovering. Or perhaps the real discovery was the anti-anxiety pill. When we were through, the technicians congratulated me on my composure.

I don't remember the wait for the scan results. It was all happening too fast. I think my anxiety reserves were all used up during the traumatic meeting with Lara.

In the world of cancer, when things take a downward turn, the decline often steepens rapidly. The MRI results were not good. What had appeared to be two discrete spots on the CT scan were actually a myriad of tiny metastases. Targeted treatment was out of the question. I would need "whole-brain radiation." The words alone horrified me, but when Karen explained the procedure, I crossed the horror barrier, just as my cancer had crossed the blood-brain barrier. I was numb.

Karen's explanation was accompanied by some demonstration pictures on her computer. First, I'd be fitted for a mask. I would lie still for half an hour or so while the mask cooled and molded to the exact shape of my head. There would be small holes for my nostrils, no opening for my mouth. There would be slits above the eyes, which would allow for partial, blurry vision. Once the mask was made, I'd have ten radiation sessions. For each one, the mask would be fitted over my face and nailed to the bed. When my head was totally immobilized and everyone had left the room, the scanner would pass over me. I'd need to take the steroid Dexamethasone daily for about three weeks. About a week after the final treatment I would lose all my hair.

And so it was. I doped myself up for the mask fitting, and I survived. I was high on Dexamethasone for all the treatments, but just to be sure, I topped up with Ativan before we set out on our daily visit to the Radiation Centre at Prince William Hospital. The actual radiation took place in the basement, a kind of modern-day chamber of horrors. The staff members were wonderful, kind, compassionate people.

I think the whole ordeal was a lot easier for me than it was for Doug. I was high. He was sober, and he had to watch. For the first time since my diagnosis, I could see that he wasn't coping. I arranged for some girlfriends to take me some of the days. They were troupers, really brave. I don't know how I would have coped if I'd had to witness such a scene.

The third day of my whole-brain radiation was also the Jewish festival of Simchat Torah. On this day we celebrate the annual cycle of Torah reading. Communities gather in their synagogues to dance in circles with their beloved Torah scrolls in their arms. Later, the very last verses of the Five Books of Moses are read from the dais, or *bimah*, and, true to the circle, we immediately move on to the beginning, when God creates the heavens and the earth. That fluent movement from end to beginning, that passing through nothing, crossing the edge, is one of the most beautiful moments in our annual cycle.

It has long been the tradition of communities to bestow special honor upon members by inviting them to recite the blessing for these two readings, and to stand at the *bimah* while the scroll is being read. He who is honored with the blessing over the last words of the Torah is called "the Groom of the Torah," and he who is honored with the blessing over the first words is called "the Groom of Genesis."

The festival of Simchat Torah comes at the end of the intense period of worship that begins with Rosh Hashanah, closely followed by Yom Kippur and Succot, the "Feast of Tabernacles." This run of so many days of prayer and contemplation heightens the wildness of the Simchat Torah celebration. The dancing is fast, abandoned, but for me, the joy is often tinged with sadness. By this point I am glad, in a way, to be returning to a normal schedule of weekdays and Sabbaths, but I am also sorry. I love the High Holy Days, they are as delicious as any spiritual retreat I can think of, and on Simchat Torah I often find myself reluctant to part from them, longing to reach back into them, to remain in those slower, quieter days of swaying and singing and praying, when time and schedules dissolve. Those are precious days. Simchat Torah marks their end, for another year. After Simchat Torah I must take that step, over the end, perhaps into the abyss, if I am to move on to the next beginning.

There's a beautiful Hassidic story about Rebbe Baruch confronting a student who, after studying too much Kabbalah for his tender years, believes he has arrived at the brink of a great abyss.

"Rebbe!" he cries. "Please help me!"

"You can't unlearn what you have already learned," the Rebbe replies. "There's only one thing to do."

"What is that, Rebbe?" the distraught student asks.

"We must move forward," says Rebbe Baruch.

"Into the abyss?" asks the student, trembling.

"Hold my hand," says Rebbe Baruch. "Let us jump together, and see if we don't land in Faith…"

That is how I feel on Simchat Torah, when we are asked to jump into the end and land in the beginning.

Our community is Orthodox, but egalitarian, meaning that we stretch women's participation in services to the limits allowed by Orthodox Jewish law. Men and women sit separately, but they sit at the same level, divided equally by a transparent curtain drawn down the middle of the room, cutting directly across the *bimah* from which the Torah is read, giving access to both men and women. Women lead parts of the services, women chant the readings from the Torah, women openly recite the mourner's Kaddish for deceased parents. Before and after the Torah reading, the holy scroll is passed through the women's section, and the women kiss it, as do the men, when it passes. These may sound like small concessions, but in the world of Orthodox Judaism they are major breakthroughs. My community suits my taste for Judaism. I find it meaningless and pasty without the beauty of its ancient rituals, but impossibly alienating if I am excluded and relegated to the role of onlooker.

And so, true to our community's values, we allow for "Brides" as well as "Grooms" on Simchat Torah.

That year, at the end of my first reprieve, I was invited to be "the Bride of the Torah," to say the blessing over its very last words. I arrived quite late, as I'd first had to report to the Radiotherapy Centre to have my head bolted to the bed and zapped. The steroids I was taking were hyping me up and messing with my head. By the time I arrived at the synagogue, the dancing had ended, and people were being "called to the Torah" to hear the opening verses of its final portion. The verses are read over and over, until every congregant has been "called up." Everyone, that is, except those two who are this year's "Bride" and "Groom."

I was too worn out and hyped up to really know what to expect. When everyone had returned to their seats and I was called up as "the Bride of the Torah," I prepared to make my way to the *bimah*, but before I could get to my feet a group of men had breached the divide and grabbed the legs of my chair, lifting me aloft over their heads.

I shrieked. I laughed. Then I cried. Then I laughed again. They danced me round to the beat of everyone clapping until my mother, who had ventured into this unfamiliar territory to watch my investiture, cried out in alarm. I was gently returned to the ground, and when I regained my land legs I stood at the *bimah* before the open scroll, next to the reader.

The young woman who was "calling me" began to recite the beautiful poetic Hebrew of the "investiture." When she read, or rather sang, "Arise, arise, Deborah, daughter of Israel, Bride of the Torah, and render honor to the great and awesome God, and in reward for this may you be deemed worthy to see children and grandchildren…" my whole body shook. From the midst of the crowd, my daughter Orly made a move toward me and, encouraged by the other women, she came to stand by me. She is so petite, my Orly, so vulnerable despite her hard shell. I cradled her in my arm, and she rested her head on my shoulder, and we cried and laughed together.

I recited the blessing, and the reader, a master of the art, began to chant the final verses of the Torah, the account of the death of Moses, who never did get to enter his Promised Land. Watching the reader touch the silver pointer to the words in the scroll as he chanted them so beautifully, I was overwhelmed by my love for this document, this text, this narrative of creation, exile, and redemption that I had read over and over, year after year, always finding newness, depth, emotion, always finding my own vagrant heart, my "unthought known" as Avivah calls it. I was never disappointed. I overflowed with love for these perfectly formed Hebrew letters, these words that flew and flamed and made my spirit soar.

Over the past year, I had taught this entire text week by week, every Thursday morning in my sunlit front room, and now I was here, standing before the actual handwritten scroll, staring through my tears at the handcrafted letters on the parchment, holding my daughter tight, at the end, and before the beginning. It was a moment of pure love.

21

That moment helped carry me through the bleak period ahead. I completed my ten days of whole-brain radiation, emerging washed out and half crazed from the steroids. As predicted, my hair began to fall from my scalp a week or so after the final session. Such a weird experience; it just disengaged, as if it had been uprooted and exiled. I could have shaved it as soon as it started to fall, but I continued to hope that some may remain, that despite the doctors' predictions, it may just thin. Perhaps I would not be entirely bald.

I wish I had shaved it. Pulling the long strands out became an obsessive occupation. For most of my life, my hair had been my glory. I was even born with a full head of it. Long, dark, almost black, with a curl and a kick, I was often described as "the one with the hair." It had been my trademark since childhood. But by the time of the brain radiation, it had thinned considerably due to the hormone-suppressing medication I'd taken during my first reprieve. I'd already lost a lot. How much more could there be?

You would be surprised how much hair can fall from a woman's head, even when it is no longer super-thick and glossy, no longer a trademark. For a week, I stood for hours each day under the shower, despite Melbourne's severe drought and water restrictions, pulling, pulling, feeling it come away in my hands, fistfuls of it, disengaging, as if it had never really been attached. And not only in the shower. I would sit for hours in my recliner chair in the kitchen, pulling, pulling, more hair, more hair. I collected it all, from the shower, from the chair, and Doug buried it in the garden. Bald patches of scalp appeared. I was losing my identity. I was a woman in transition.

Finally, my scalp was smooth and unshadowed. I was completely bald. My eyebrows and eyelashes mostly went too. When I stared at the strange face in the mirror, the unframed eyes seemed continually startled; the animal caught in the headlights. I was surprised to find that my scalp was not rounded, not really symmetrical at all, and it came to a kind of Martian-looking point at the top.

I'd always hated covering my hair. Hats and scarves brought out the claustrophobic in me, but now I would have to adapt.

A wig. Yes, a wig! My friend Rita drove me to one of the most stylish and expensive wig-makers in the city. This was a private appointment. I was alone with Chaya, the Orthodox Jewish wig-maker, and Rita, my Swiss-Jewish friend, and for the first time, I exposed my new head in front of others. Even Doug had not yet seen my bald pate. I wore a small cap to bed, and a scarf during the day. I thought I'd feel safe with Rita and Chaya. Rita is such a close friend, and hugely compassionate, and Chaya has the distinction of having the most children of anyone I know. (I think the last count was seventeen.) I just hadn't realized how traumatizing, how humiliating this would be. I'd thought of it as a small inconvenience, something to be overlooked in the big picture. I'd convinced myself that losing my hair would mean little to me. But removing the scarf in front of those women, kind and caring as they were, was tough. Looking back, I can see that I had not really thought things through.

Chaya pulled some wigs out of the rack, and then I saw it – a replica of my own hair! It was perfect! It was human hair, incredibly expensive, but it was *my* hair, exactly. What I failed to see was that it *was* my hair, as it had been when I was thirty. I was a woman of fifty now. And I refused to register how uncomfortable the wig felt when it was on my head, how strange, how alien. No. I wanted that wig. All I could see was myself again. It would take some adjustments, some trimming, but I could get myself back. That wig would be my hair, and I would no longer be bald. I would have my trademark back. I would not have to adjust to this new persona. Everything would be just as it was.

I bought the wig impulsively, frantically, and returned home triumphant. Of course I never wore it, not once. It hurt my head. It looked silly, a young woman's mane framing a middle-aged chemo-drawn face. The wig was a very expensive fantasy. It was fairy-floss, an empty dream. It sat in my room on its stand for two years, until finally I gave it away to an ultra-Orthodox woman, a mother of ten, whose strict standards of modesty demanded that her hair be covered at all times. Never in her married life had she been able to afford a real human-hair wig.

I often wondered about the original owner of that hair. I imagined a beautiful, upright, brown-skinned woman sunk in poverty somewhere in Asia, or maybe South America, who grew her hair for sale, like wheat or corn, to buy food for her children. Owning her hair, touching it, had felt like an intimacy I had not been permitted.

My oncologist had predicted that my hair regrowth would be delayed due to the chemo that was to follow the brain radiation, but that it would return, probably in three to six months. She was wrong. A year later, I am still waiting, It has regrown in places, but the crown is still completely bare. Apparently this happens in a small minority of cases. I've been told that at this point regrowth is highly unlikely. I am stuck with my bald pate.

I have more or less learned the art of the head-scarf, and it *is* an art. People say I look good in scarves. I choose to believe them, although when I look in the mirror, I'm not so sure. When I look in the mirror, I'm not sure about anything. I've collected many scarves. I dress to match them, my silky scarves, with long tassels hanging down the back, and fringes on the sides like colorful hair, like a rasta woman. I have, I suppose, grown accustomed to my scarves. They are my trademark. I am "the one with the head-scarves." A whole new me.

I was given just two weeks to get body and soul into some sort of order after the twenty-first-century horrors of whole-brain radiation, and then it was back to Day Oncology at St. Katherine's. I was still whacked out from the radiation, but I couldn't wait any longer for chemo. The tumors in my lungs were growing. Nothing was easy. Lara decided to put me back on Taxotere, because it had worked so well on me the first time around. I couldn't fault her reasoning. Why start plundering the breast cancer treatment pharmacy before we have to?

This time, instead of eight weekly sessions, I was to have four heavy-dose sessions at three-week intervals. The first session knocked me out for the count. For the first two weeks I could to nothing but lie in bed or on my recliner chair and try not to cry. I was still reeling and exhausted from the brain zapping. The Taxotere made me nauseous and horribly flat, moodless. I ached all over. I lost my taste for vegetables, for soup, for fruit, even for water! Toast, cookies, and chocolate became my staple. The very thought of water made my stomach turn. The very life force, the greatest treasure known to humankind, repulsed me. It was midsummer in Melbourne. Dehydrated and sickened by the thought of clear fresh water, I took to sucking popsicles and popping pieces of ice in my mouth.

The chemo was poisoning my mind. It was turning me against my greatest allies. Doris made me a tape in which she attempted to convince me that the chemo was my friend. I listened to it, nearly every night. I knew the power of chemo. I hoped it would save my life. I willed it to. I imagined the chemo making its way into my lungs, annihilating the rebel cells, crunching them underfoot. I was grateful to the chemo for the job it was capable of doing, but I couldn't love it. How could I? It didn't love me. It hurt me deeply, and worse, it refused to cross the blood-brain barrier and attack the rebels in my brain. What's the use of a body without a head?

I knew it could be saving me, but I felt as if it was killing me as well. Chemo is indiscriminate. It crushes everything underfoot. It is a great jackboot, a brute that destroys everything in its path and leaves behind it smoking, scorched earth.

This time around, the chemo hit me harder and landed me in hospital twice. A few days after the second of the four treatments, my temperature soared, and I was rushed to the St. Katherine's Emergency Room with plummeting white blood cells. After taking a blood test, the doctor wryly informed me I had *no* white blood cells. I had severe neutropenia, and was open to any passing infection. Great time to be lying in an open emergency room, but there were no beds available on the ward. I was tucked away in a quiet corner, left with Doug and told to wait. Much later, in the middle of the night, an orderly approached our corner.

"He's coming to tell us they've found a private room!" I said, trying to keep my sense of humor.

"Madame," he said, sounding French. "We have found you a private room."

Now that is light in the heart of darkness! That's what salvation's all about!

I was happy in my little corner room, near where Ben had been, with a lovely view of the mountains and good meals served regularly. I rested and read. I was being fed antibiotics through a drip and recovered within a few days.

All in all, it could have been a lot worse – and it was, the next time I was hospitalized. I spent half the night in Emergency, and then with peaking fever, attached to a drip, suffering violent episodes of diarrhea, and vulnerable to any passing infections, I was moved to a four-bed ward. I was prioritized for a private room, but none were available.

Two of the four beds were next to the window. One faced the door, and mine faced the bathroom. That was my entire view, for almost a week, and I wasn't the only one in the ward with chemo-induced diarrhea.

When I arrived, the women in the three other beds were receiving chemo treatments as inpatients. This was often an option for people having chemo for the first time, especially if they were worried about coping alone at home for the first night. I was the only one being treated for neutropenia. I shouldn't have been there. I wanted a private room, but it was the holiday season, the oncology ward was overbooked and understaffed, and there was not a single room to be had. So I lay in the four-bed ward, staring at the bathroom door. If the door was left open, as it often was, I had a direct view of the toilet.

I lay in bed, attached to my drip. My artist friend Jane arrived one afternoon and took pictures of me and "Drip," my new lover. Jane decorated us with flowers, I put my arm around Drip, and held signs saying "I've got you under my skin." It was fun for a moment. But this time the fever wouldn't abate, and mostly I was miserable, truly miserable. In that noisy, close, four-bed ward I was forced to admit my JAPdom. Yes, somewhere along the road of life I had become a Jewish Australian Princess. I don't think I was born that way. I can recall proudly enduring much tougher conditions in my younger years. JAPdom had been thrust upon me by the responsibilities of wifedom and motherhood, and especially by the demands of illness, and my growing sense of myself as fragile, as precious.

Having no alternative, I remained feverish and miserable in the four-bed ward, and watched the passing parade.

The night I arrived, the woman in the bed directly opposite mine was not happy. She called for the nurse about every half-hour. The site where her UV drip had been attached was aching. She felt dizzy. Her toes felt numb. I felt for her. Chemo is a scary experience. You have no idea what it's doing to you, and every strange feeling becomes exaggerated and seems life-threatening. In the morning, the woman's daughter came to take her home. She had yet to look at me directly, but as she left on her daughter's arm, she glanced at me. I couldn't make out her expression.

Her replacement more than made up for the earlier occupant's reticence. A very hefty, newly diagnosed Jewish woman, she eschewed her bed and settled herself in a visitor's chair, from which she regaled me, for hours, with the by now two-week-old story of her breast cancer diagnosis. I felt for her too. I could see she was still in shock. She was alone, she said, no husband, no children, although I did learn later of a flock of devoted siblings, nieces, and nephews. But she was frightened and feeling sorry for herself. She'd recovered well from the mastectomy, and was due for follow-up chemo. She'd opted to stay overnight in hospital for her first chemo session, as she was afraid of possible reactions and wanted to be monitored. Fair enough. It's not that I resented her two-week-old story of early breast cancer. I wished her well, I really did, but a year and a half down the track, with stage-four incurable cancer, I just didn't want to hear it. I was envious. It's not nice to say, but I was.

She was a nice woman, warm, and obese. I could see that she hated her girth, that it tormented her. She was continually running herself down, making fun of her fat. The nurses had trouble fitting a blood-pressure cuff on her, even the larger size, the one made for legs. When they squeezed it tight, it kept popping off. The woman was just too large. After a while, my envy disappeared. She talked incessantly of her health, not just about recent events, but her entire medical history. In my former life I would have dismissed her as a raving hypochondriac, but in recent times, as I learned more about the human predicament, I had become a little more openhearted. When she left the ward the following day in a wheelchair that the nurse insisted she didn't need, complaining of heartburn after eating two breakfasts in a row, I felt affection for her, and even some love. Her niece, a pretty curly-topped girl, had come to collect her. When she left she waved from her wheelchair, reminding me of the Queen. I wished her well, and I meant it.

The four-bed-ward experience became more interesting, and horrific, as the days went by. Despite my pleas, my tears, my raging fever, my diarrhea, no private room was available. I was a JAP stuck in the trenches, with only the toilet for diversion. It was terrible, but it was also becoming difficult to ignore the humorous side.

My next roommate, given the bed diagonally opposite mine, under the window, was a middle-aged woman in an immaculate figure-hugging power suit who was brought in kicking and screaming early one morning, clutching her laptop.

"This is a mistake!" she yelled. "I came to see Dr. Browne because I was just a bit dizzy. I was just checking in. I'm not supposed to be here. I'm due at a meeting!"

"Your blood pressure is very low. You'll have to wait here now until Dr. Browne signs your release. He's waiting to see if you need further tests." The nurse was formal, but not unkind.

The woman lay on her bed in her power suit, refusing to get under the covers. She pulled out a mobile phone.

"Darling. They've kidnapped me. Yes, I'm at the hospital, in a ward. You're going to have to go ahead without me. Of course I'm all right. It's just a stupid mix-up. I'm fine. I was a bit dizzy, is all, probably a side effect of my meds. Now they're doing a bloody battery of unnecessary tests." She coughed, and I noticed how pale she was, and I noticed the dark rings around her eyes. They could have been the smudges of mascara, but they weren't.

In the Book of Exodus, Pharaoh would not let the Israelites go. It didn't matter what the world hit him with, it didn't matter how much devastation, flood, or pestilence, how many locusts or boils, he refused to face facts. He insisted on carrying on, as if nothing were happening.

Denial, says Rabbi Hoffman, is a river in Egypt.

Then there was the little old woman who took the bed next to mine, the one under the window that I so, so coveted. She was a small, bent woman, and she arrived on the arm of a small, bent man. They spoke English to each other, with Viennese accents. He settled her into bed, carefully, asking questions to which she mumbled replies, and then he walked up and down our tiny ward, cracking jokes. His wife was a little demented, so she mostly ignored him. They were obviously Jewish: the banter, the jokes, the worn faces, and the depth in their eyes, what else could they be? So when the little man approached my bed, I called him with a welcoming gesture and wished him a happy Hanukkah.

He clutched the rail of my bed. He even unbent a little. He looked me straight in the eye.

"What are you talking about?" he snapped, lowering his voice to a whisper. "What is Hanukkah? I don't know what you're talking about!"

I apologized. He walked away, quickly, back to his slightly demented wife. When he was ready to leave her for the night, when he had tucked her in and planted a sweet wet kiss on her forehead, he crept back to my bed.

"How did you know?" he whispered, urgently, in his Jewish Viennese accent. "No one is supposed to know. When we came to this country we dropped all of that. It only ever brought us trouble. A Jew? I am not a Jew! I am an Australian. I am safe." He looked at me, sadly, a memory fluttering in his eyes. I could see in their depths the Hanukkah candles lit at eventide by the window, and him as a boy standing with the family that was gone, all gone up in smoke.

"Happy Hanukkah," he whispered. I could barely make out the words, and he rushed out of the room.

All night his tiny, fragile wife called out. She couldn't figure out how to use the nurse-call button, so she just cried out, over and over.

"Help me! Help me! I need the toilet."

I pressed my nurse-call button. When the nurse arrived, I directed her to the next bed.

An hour later, another call.

"Help! Help me. Please. Somebody help me! I need to roll over!"

Again I pressed the button, again I redirected the nurse. All night it went on, at regular intervals, as my fever rose, and rose. By morning, I was burning up, drenched in sweat. I called for the nurse, who arrived swiftly and walked right past my bed, ignoring me, to tend to my elderly Viennese neighbor. She was sleeping peacefully. Finally, the nurse got to me. I had to laugh.

The funniest and the saddest roommate of all was the woman who on my final day in the ward replaced the Viennese lady.

She arrived full of beans, carrying her bag, chatting away to anyone who would listen. She was in for three days, she said, and would receive a slow-drip chemo the entire time. This was her second session. She'd lost over twenty kilos since the last one, she told me with pride.

"How did you manage that?" I asked.

"I forgot to stock up on food before I got sick on chemo. By then I was too weak to go to the shops. So I didn't eat. I just watched the telly." She spoke cheerily.

"Don't you have anyone to help you?" I asked.

"Nope," she answered, as if this was the most natural thing in the world. "The council worker stopped by, nice girl, but I wasn't up to chatting. Nope. It's just me, myself, and I."

As it happened, Lara was her oncologist as well. When she arrived on her rounds, she pulled the curtain around my neighbor's bed, but I couldn't help overhearing the conversation.

"You'll be weak when you leave here in three days," said Lara. "Do you have someone picking you up?"

"Nope. I'll get the bus, like last time."

"How far is it from the bus stop to your flat?"

"Aw, about fifteen minutes."

"Is there no one to pick you up?"

"Nah. I'll be right. I learned my lesson. This time I'll buy food on the way home and put it in the freezer. I've got the telly. I'll be right."

How could she do it? How could she face it all alone? Just her and the TV.

She clammed up after Lara's visit. I guess the chemo was starting to get to her. Instead of her chatter I was treated to her TV, at full volume, tuned to the tennis. She lay there for hours, egging on the players, swearing at them, occasionally roaring, although I couldn't figure out why. I think she just forgot that there were others in the room. When the tennis ended she flicked channels, late into the night. Now and then she'd comment loudly on what she was viewing. She didn't turn the telly off and she didn't turn herself off. I guess that's how she got by alone at home.

The following afternoon, I reached breaking point. I had decided to check myself out, fever and all, but God intervened. It was Friday evening. Sari, my friend and GP, had come with Orly to share a Sabbath evening meal with me. We found a quiet place in the corridor, near the lifts. I brought Drip along, of course. The nurses were cooperative. One stopped by to take my temperature. Still too high, but the thought of returning to that crazy ward after the meal was over sent chills right through me.

And then the miracle happened.

My nurse reappeared. A woman in a small private room had become unexpectedly violent. The staff couldn't handle her, and her son had been called to take her home. The room would be ready in an hour, and it was mine.

The room was mine! A few years back, how could I have imagined such delight at such a turn of events? My appetite returned, I enjoyed the meal, and we waited out the hour in the corridor. When we were told the room was ready I grabbed Drip and moved faster than I had in months. Sari and Orly dragged behind, laughing. I never looked back. I went straight to my room. My room! Sari and Orly collected my things from the ward. I never went back. But I do think about the woman and her telly. And sometimes I think of the others I met in there.

If I'd retained the desire of my younger, less troubled days, the desire to write short stories that others may like to read, or at least stories that I imagined others may like to read, I might have got a bit of mileage out of my time in the ward. But I've passed that place, for the moment anyway. I'm writing for myself, not to please others. The ward was a nightmare.

22

I loved my new room. It was small and opposite the main reception desk, so not all that quiet, but it was mine, my own space, a place where I could return to myself and take stock.

My fever finally vanished, and I began to read, to enjoy my visitors, to look forward to going home. But the big question remained – what to do about the chemo? I couldn't go on like this, showing up at Emergency with neutropenia a week after every session. Lara arranged for me to have a CT scan to assess the state of my lungs before suggesting another strategy.

I was wheeled down for the scan in my dressing gown, as an inpatient, and waited with others in a special secluded area, for my turn. The CT went smoothly, and I was wheeled back to my room by a young guy, a budding sportsman, who admitted to treating our journey down the hospital hallways as training for a forthcoming race. I enjoyed speeding. It was fun, but when I saw the flash of a familiar face as we whizzed by, I held up my arm, like a charioteer, and called a halt.

It was Alana, a member of my spiritual community, a lovely girl with a beautiful voice, a fledgling career as a performance artist, and an almost completed medical degree. She promised to visit me later in the day.

And she did, with some interesting information. When I told her about the Taxotere and the recurrent neutropenia, she asked why I hadn't had "the injection."

"What injection?" I asked.

"The one they give everyone after chemo, as a matter of course, to boost their white blood cells."

"No one ever offered me one. It's the first I've heard of it."

Alana's mother had been treated for early breast cancer the previous year, and had received "the injection" after each of her designated treatments.

We were both perplexed. I agreed to ask Lara about it when she stopped by with the scan results during her evening rounds.

I was alone when Lara arrived. Doug had gone out for a walk. She was wearing her serious face. I squirmed. The first set of news was not bad. The lung lesions had remained stable. No shrinkage, but no significant progression, either. The measurements had increased slightly, but the increase remained within the statistical margin of error.

"Stable is good," said Lara, "but we'll have to think about moving you onto another treatment. The Taxotere is sending you into hospital every time, and you can't go on like this."

I asked her about "the injection."

Lara looked uncomfortable. I think her cheeks even colored a little. "It's only free for patients with early-stage disease. You'd have to pay."

"How much?"

"Three thousand dollars a pop."

I tried to get my head around that. Free for those with early disease, free as a matter of course. They didn't have to wind up in hospital with neutropenia even once. They got the injection as a precaution, just in case.

I'd been hospitalized twice, I obviously needed the injection, yet still I didn't qualify.

Ah. It fell into place. Adjuvant therapy, "clean-up chemo" used for cases caught early, was administered for a definitive amount of time, and then it ended. Advanced cases like mine could have many, many rounds of chemo, with no end in sight. The financial burden was too great. I decided to ignore, for the time being, the consideration that it might not be considered financially viable to give such an expensive drug to "incurables." The very fact that had once sunk me into a slough of despond now lifted my spirits. I can't have it for free because they're banking on me being here for a long, long while. Wonderful! Bring it on! That's what I like to hear. It totally compensated for my private health fund, which had agreed to allow me to move up to top-level coverage, despite my pre-existing disease, on condition that I paid now and waited one year for the new benefits to take effect. I guessed, from a financial standpoint, they were banking on me not being around to collect.

But the government had faith in me! They wouldn't give me "the injection" because I might stubbornly hang around, way past my use-by date, and cost them too much. Wonderful!

I turned to Lara. "Lara," I said, "I know that Doug and I look like destitute hippies, and I guess I act like one, but I need you to know that my mother has money, and she is prepared to spend whatever it takes. Please, please, inform me of all my options."

It was the first really proactive move I'd made all by myself since my initial diagnosis. I was moving toward taking some responsibility for the steps of this journey. It was a good moment. I think that Lara felt it too.

"I'd like to complete the final rounds of Taxotere," I said, "but with the injection. We'll pay."

I did complete them, and we never did pay. Duncan, a kindly, righteous soul in the hospital pharmacy, talked the pharmacist into giving me samples recently sent by the drug company. At the time, it felt like a miracle, not because of the money saved, but because of Duncan's kindness.

I wish my bedside meeting with Lara could have ended there, on the high note, with me feeling empowered and even perhaps a little in control. But that look returned to Lara's face, especially in her eyes. Concerned, they were. Concerned.

"Debbie, something else came up on the scan."

I'd learned a few things about Lara. When she used my name, I generally had to brace myself.

"They've picked up a few spots on your bones, small spots. One on the sternum, one on the right hip, and one above the pubic bone.

I closed my eyes. "It's spread to my bones? Are they sure?"

"It's not likely to be anything else, Debbie. The spots didn't show on earlier scans, so they are probably not scar tissue from some past injuries. They are new developments. It has all the hallmarks of metastasized cancer. But we won't confirm it until you've had a bone scan. I've arranged one for tomorrow."

And on it goes. Doug returned. Lara patiently re-explained the "developments." I was silent, on the outside. Inside, I was busy with my questions.

Okay. So now you have breast cancer which has spread to your lungs, your brain and...your bones. I felt tears prick my eyes. Inside. My bones? It's in my bones? The prophets had fire in their bones, and I have cancer? Where's the sense in that? Where's the God in that? Where is God? Where are You? Show Yourself! Not in the bones! The bones hold me together. What do You want from me?

"Bone metastases are very manageable," Lara was saying. "And these are very small. We'll just add Zometa, a bone strengthener, you can have it after your regular Herceptin infusion. There are a few side effects to Zometa, but I don't think that the mets themselves are going to cause you much trouble. Of all the possible metastases, they are the most manageable."

I later learned that she was correct. Those with advanced breast cancer that had spread only to the bones live longer, statistically that is.

But back then, I hadn't done the research, and I didn't believe her. All I knew was that the cancer was spreading, and I was terrified. It all seemed so hopeless.

I remained quiet. I don't think that Lara or Doug saw the extent of my terror. When they had gone, I turned out the light and lay in the dark, crying. I was back in the Book of Psalms.

Put my tears in Your bottle: they are already in Your book.

Some time during the night a nurse entered, shining a flashlight, to take my temperature. She was not my favorite nurse. I found her brusque, and her torch was invasive. But when her flashlight picked up my tears, she put away her log book and pulled up a chair.

I told her what was going on, how helpless I felt.

She responded in a strong, certain voice, as if she'd been through this before, and of course she had. She was a nurse on the oncology ward. And so she spoke, a set piece, probably, telling me everything I didn't want to hear.

"Get a blank sheet of paper," she advised. "Write down everything you want to do, and do it. Like pulling wishes out of a bucket. One by one, fulfill all your wishes."

She was predicting my early death, telling me to cram everything in while I still had time. She reduced me to some make-a-wish bucket case. I didn't want to hear that. I wanted to hear about how I was going to get through this, and see my children marry, and know my children's children. And she was advising me in the middle of the night on how to prepare to die.

And yet, strangely, I was comforted. I guess all I needed was a voice in the night. Even one that was telling me that I was a done deal.

23

It's hard to imagine, but other stories were afoot in my life at this time, or perhaps they are all strands of the same story. As time passes, as I write it all out of me, I tend toward the latter. I doubt I'll ever see all the strands, no matter how close I come, and I doubt I'll ever see the big picture, no matter how much distance I get. But my sense of it is there, and growing as I write.

Between my bouts in and out of hospital, between the chemo sessions and the existential encounters with mortality, I was bringing a book into the world. Yes, a book!

Some years earlier, before my initial diagnosis, Avivah Zornberg had surprised me in one of her weekly letters by suggesting I try my hand at writing. She knew I was a writer. I'd written a couple of novels, some magazine features, and short stories, some of which I was pleased with and some of which had pleased her. But this was a whole other ballpark. Avivah was talking about writing Torah. She was encouraging me to join a great and daunting chain of Torah scholars who actually felt that they had some new, novel, enlightening take on our ancient text.

I was moved by her confidence and her enthusiasm, but I also seriously wondered if she had weighed her words. During the first few years of our weekly correspondence I had become a competent teacher of Torah. I could manipulate and sometimes illuminate texts and their commentaries in ways that often inspired students to look at their own lives and interactions through the prism of the Torah's wisdom. In preparing my weekly *parshah* classes I'd spend hours combing through the commentaries of the masters, looking for glimmers of some new connection, some uplifting resonance. Rarely, very rarely, perhaps once or twice a year, I stumbled upon something that might actually point to some new direction.

This was far from "Torah scholarship." *I* was far from Torah scholarship, not only because I had so much to learn, but because at that stage of my life, I couldn't bear the thought of uncertainty. Every strain of narrative in the Torah needed meaning, and not only meaning, but meaning that connected directly to higher meaning, and so forth, all the way to a great unified meaning, a great closure. If I could teach a class where every pretty thread tied neatly to another, giving us in the end the vision of a big beautiful bow, all across the cosmos, then I would be happy with a job well done.

So Avivah suggested I try my hand at writing. Okay. First thing, then, to my mind, was to find my Grand Unifying Story. Looking back from this more distant future, I can see Avivah chuckling. The unity came naturally to my mind, which had never craved anything but. I decided to divide my Torah commentary into a great cycle of creation, fragmentation, exile, and redemption, basically allowing the stories of Genesis and Exodus to tell the whole human saga.

I divided my four great mystical moments into chapters and wrote an outline for each chapter.

Torah scholarship was easy! I sat at my desk and wrote and wrote and within a few months I had about forty thousand words! Having read and reread Avivah's two groundbreaking works on Genesis and Exodus, I had her style down pat. My writing was eloquent, subtle, finely wrought. One could barely hear a trace of anything but a poor imitation of Avivah in it.

I sent it to her as a file attachment to an email, and waited one, two, three days. Longer than I expected. The reply, when it finally came, hit me in the guts, a metal bullet of truth that cut right into me.

The world doesn't need another potted history of Kabbalah, she wrote, kindly omitting that even if it did, there were many more qualified than I to do it. Even more kindly, she omitted to mention that the world doesn't need another Avivah Zornberg wannabe.

As I reread my work through the prism of her criticism, I saw that this was exactly what I had been trying to do. Trying not to feel humiliated of course increased my sense of shame, but to my credit, I stopped blocking it, allowed myself to feel it, and was able to move on. I was even able to laugh a little.

One of Avivah's most remarkable characteristics is her capacity for compassionate fellowship. In her quiet, confident, and enthusiastic way, she was encouraging me to find my own voice. She never tried to steer me into a particular direction, she never offered suggestions. She just walked alongside me, and smiled and watched. Later, when she launched the book that I finally wrote under her gentle tutelage, I was amazed to discover how much she had learned about the discovery of voice and the process required to achieve it, just by watching me, and smiling.

After the failure of a second forty-thousand-word attempt at "learned" verbosity, I was ready to give up. I had no formal Jewish education. I could barely read and understand the text in the original. What did I have to offer? Okay, I could inspire people in my neighborhood to look more deeply into their own lives, but how could that translate into something of literary or scholarly merit? I let the whole thing go. And yet, beneath my consciousness, I was completely engaged in the process, as Avivah understood it.

The first time I heard the poetry of the great Indian Nobel laureate Rabindranath Tagore, it was from Avivah.

On the seashore of endless worlds, children play.

Drawing on the research of the English psychoanalyst Donald Winnicott, Avivah used this quote from Tagore to illustrate the concept of "doodle time," of the empty spaces we need in our lives and in our thoughts, if living waters are to have any hope of springing forth from some long-buried source.

I had never been good at making space. I was a proud multitasker. I even wanted my dreams to be useful, to serve some conscious daytime goal. Yet my soul understood Avivah's teaching, which was for me at the very heart of the Jewish mystical tradition that I so loved. Without void, without emptiness, nothing is created, nothing is creatable. Fashioning elaborate book plans with all the spaces already filled in was not a way to find a voice. Finding a voice involved hesitation, uncertainty, a sense of powerlessness and absence. If I had a voice, I had not yet discovered it. If it was there at all it was deep within. I could stamp my feet and command it to appear, but that of course would be futile.

I gave up writing projects and continued to teach. Once in a while, I wrote a short, pithy piece for Melbourne's Sunday newspaper, for a column called "Faith." I wrote about Jewish festivals from a mystical perspective, and the newspaper published them on the Sunday of the week in which they were celebrated. I earned a bit of money, but I didn't consider it "real" writing.

Then came an email from Mark, the president of our spiritual community. He wanted to send an e-letter to all the congregants each week, to encourage them to come to the Sabbath services. Would I contribute a very short piece on the weekly Torah reading, say 350 words?

"C'mon Deb," he wrote. "It's nothing to you. You could do it with your eyes closed, and you'll be helping the community."

This was before my diagnosis, when I never said no.

Despite my frantic timetable, I got to work. That week's reading was about the spies sent ahead to scout the Promised Land, the very same reading that a year later would give me some comfort amid the trauma of diagnosis. It was all about doubt and vision.

I didn't look up a lot of sources. I wrote from the top of my head, and what came out was a sort of prose poem, a playing with words and concepts backed up by what I already knew from the various commentaries. It was fun. The prose was there in the story, which I loved as much as anything, and the poetry was in my obsessive desire to stay within the word limit.

I wrote week after week, allowing an idea to arise, usually in the shower or on a walk. I'd write the piece, then spend an entire day honing it, word by word, as if I were shaping a sculpture, or arranging flowers.

I was a child playing on the shores of endless worlds, and I did not know it. I didn't think about what I was doing, I just did it, because it was fun.

A month or so later, I set out on my fateful pilgrimage to Safed, to study with Rabbi Hoffman. Before traveling to Safed, I spent a few days in Jerusalem with my sister Aviva and her family, and one evening, of course, I visited Avivah Zornberg. This was only our second face-to-face meeting, but we'd been corresponding weekly for years. The face-to-face awkwardness I'd feared dissolved within a few minutes. I still find it hard to believe, but there is some kind of true kinship between Avivah and me that actually succeeds in conquering our mutual and quite intense shyness. We are able to open up to each other, not on the surface but from the depths, within minutes.

During the course of the evening, Avivah spoke to me about voice in a way that helped me to believe, maybe for the first time in my life, that I might actually have one. When we parted, I handed her a few examples of the prose poems I'd been writing and a few of the pieces I'd written for the Sunday newspaper.

She went to America and I went to Safed. When I returned to Australia after running away from the bombs, I received an email from her telling me that she thought perhaps I had found my voice.

I spent another few years working on the prose poems. During the first year I wrote weekly, until I had covered every reading in the Torah, and the second year, the year of my initial diagnosis, I edited everything that I'd written. Throughout those two years I only worked on pieces during the week they were read out in the synagogue. I wrote pieces for the newspaper on every festival and fast day. I had a book! I had a voice!

During the first year of writing I applied for a grant from an American foundation.

As I suspect is the case with the great majority of inexperienced grant applicants, I thought it was in the bag. I filled out the forms. My work in progress seemed exactly the sort of thing they were looking to fund. I needed three referees. Mark, a respected academic, wrote a glowing recommendation. Sam Lipski, well known in the worlds of publishing and Jewish philanthropy, contributed a page that made me blush, and, to cap it off, Avivah, a world-renowned Torah scholar, gave it high praise. The grant was in the bag. It was just a matter of waiting, and as I waited, I kept writing.

Why did I want a grant? I'm not really sure. I didn't really need the money. I could have managed without it. I guess I wanted it because it would give my work value. I pictured my publication, with the details of the grant on the back cover. A grant from an international foundation meant that my writing was worth something. And that meant that I was worth something.

By the time the letter finally arrived, I'd been diagnosed with advanced breast cancer. My application was rejected, and really, it was no big deal. That's probably the best way to explain the effect of incurable cancer on my life. The diagnosis didn't just affect my life; it affected my entire understanding of life. My whole notion of what was important was fundamentally altered. Life became a large panorama, and truth became something hidden, pure, connected to a source that had nothing to do with worth or acceptance.

I threw the letter away and kept writing. A few months later, I realized that although I really cared not a whit about a rejection that once would have gnawed at my soul, I did need to inform my referees. I'd been writing to Avivah weekly, as always, but had been so uncharacteristically unconcerned by the rejection that I'd forgotten to mention it to her. I informed all three referees by email, and within minutes of sending, I received a reply from Sam.

"They're idiots," he wrote. "We'll fund it."

"We" was the Pratt Foundation, of which Sam was chief executive officer. Now applying for a grant from the Pratt Foundation, a huge patron of the arts, is quite a business. It would have entailed even more hard labor than I'd invested in the rejected application to the American foundation. I'd never thought of asking, and it fell into my lap. Did it matter? I suppose the answer is yes. Looking back without the ego-colored glasses I can see that a book of prose poems on the weekly Torah portion was unlikely to excite any publisher, anywhere. Without Sam's offer my book would probably never have seen the light of day.

As it was, the process of finding a publisher and overseeing the publication became a pleasant distraction, a sparkle of light during those dark times after the end of my first reprieve. Head masks, whole-brain radiation, nausea, chemo, hospitals, exhaustion, fear – all this was punctuated now and then by the choice of a cover, the design of a page, a list of acknowledgments.

That's how it goes in this dappled world. The longer I last, the more I see it. A mysterious world, full of suffering and injustice, sprinkled with little moments of light. The longer I last, the less important I feel, the more I see myself as a little wriggle, a pleasant but minuscule warp in a huge unfathomable scenario, whose years are significant, equally significant, be they fifty or a hundred and fifty.

I find it strange to believe in God in a world where many lives are barely lived, where catastrophes make no sense, where any attempt to superimpose a universal scheme is doomed to be ridiculous. And yet I do. I do believe. The more I fade into insignificance, the more I believe. I can't explain it, but there it is.

24

My fever abated after a week, and I was discharged from hospital, together with my brand-new bone metastases. I ditched the metaphorical wish bucket that the night nurse had given me. I was by no means ready, back then, to be counting the end of my days.

But when you're up, you're up, and when you're down, you're basically flushed down the gurgler. A week later a brain MRI revealed two lesions on the cerebellum, probably reduced but not eradicated by the whole-brain radiation. So it was back to the state-of-the-art total-care torture rack at the Prince William Hospital. Such a paradoxical place, where people were strapped to tables and zapped with the most sincere compassion, precision, love, and hope.

This time I needed targeted radiation, a process called "stereotactic surgery." A new mask was made, I got a new tape from Doris, and new phobias were conquered.

I can't remember how many zaps I had, perhaps only one. I do remember it taking a very, very long time. I remember breathing inside the mask, and making a world for myself in there. After the radiation, I remember receiving a letter from the radio-oncolcogist requesting a follow-up MRI in four months, which would be "early in the new year." I decided to sidestep the whole issue, and hope for the best.

Since I'd been diagnosed with brain metastases I'd realized that my illness had become a battle on two fronts. The first front was south of my neck. The tumors in my breast, lungs, and bones could be treated with chemo, and I had a whole pharmacy of alternatives still at my disposal. North of the neck, however, was another country.

No known chemo could break through the "blood-brain barrier." My brain metastases could be treated only through radiation or surgery. Radiation could not be repeated on the same site.

Periodically, I'd hear a distant voice deep inside, trying to communicate something. It sounded like a cold echo calling from an underground cave. "There's no such thing as a body without a head," it said. And of course I knew this to be true. I had become a living duality: a person of two interdependent lives, struggling to survive. If one collapsed, the other would follow, and yet each needed a completely different kind of care.

Meanwhile, south of the border I survived the two final rounds of chemo with the aid of "the injection." My lung and bone metastases had stabilized, but none had shrunk. Lara decided it was time to try a new drug. I switched to an oral chemo, Xeloda. I still needed to show up at Day Oncology every three weeks for my Herceptin and, since the bone met diagnosis, for Zometa, but this new chemo was taken orally. That in itself felt like a minor reprieve. Six pills a day, at meal times. I was chronically tired, a little nauseated. My nails became brittle and my feet were raw, but I still fared much better than I had on the Taxotere.

Three months later, scans revealed incredible, miraculous healing in lungs, bones, and breast. A second reprieve, and my book was ready to roll!

As I write, I hear the rattle of the roller coaster.

My family was ecstatic with the good news. I decided to shelve my concerns regarding the brain metastases and enjoy my chemo break. Three months with only Herceptin, Zoleda, Pristiq, Femara, and sleeping pills jumping around my insides, but no outright poison! Just a week after taking my last dose of chemo I began to feel better.

The timing could not have been more perfect. We had our publisher and our book. The date for the launch was approaching, and in the interim, I had a couple of pre-launch gigs lined up.

The first was at the Jewish Museum, a musical evening featuring the poetry of "Torah-Loving Troubadours." I'd invited three friends who also studied Torah and wrote poetry to join me, along with Adam Starr, a jazz musician. Sam Lipski had done everything he could to make my book impressive. He'd even arranged for a CD of selected readings to be inserted inside the back cover. The pieces were read by

Rachael Kohn, a well-known radio presenter whose lilting voice is one of the most musical I've ever heard. Adam had composed the accompanying music, and we'd spent a day putting the CD together. After a few hours with Rachael I was reminded of how it had been to make a new friend in my youth, how special friendships could be forged in the first hours of meeting.

I've always felt that my prose poems are best appreciated when read aloud. I love reading them and I love listening to Rachael reading them. Whenever I read those poems aloud, I hear my voice, the voice that was buried for so long, and I rejoice. The poetry of my three friends that evening at the museum was superbly resonant. There was nothing superficial about it. I felt as if I had entered some kind of "zone of truth," a place where the artificial and the superficial could not survive. It was a wonderful evening.

The other gig was in Sydney, at a three-day festival of Jewish learning. It was not quite as authentic for me as the reading at the Jewish Museum, but nonetheless I enjoyed it, simply because I love reading my pieces aloud. I feel that they were made for that.

The organizers of the Sydney festival had booked a luxury apartment for Doug and me, overlooking the Harbour Bridge. I felt pampered, and I loved every moment. My chemo vacation was barely underway and already I was wringing as much fun as I could out of it. Yes, I could definitely get used to these reprieves. We took walks, ate meals, watched DVDs. By the time we returned to Melbourne, I was refreshed and ready to march into the book launch.

Some months earlier my friend Chooch had come up with a plan to bring Avivah Zornberg to Melbourne for the launch. As a result, the Centre for Jewish Civilization, of which our mutual friend Mark was director, invited Avivah to give a series of lectures and master classes at Monash University, and my book launch was scheduled to coincide with her visit. I was incredibly moved by Chooch's initiative and by Avivah's willingness to travel so far. I was aware that all this "special treatment" – the luxury apartment in Sydney, the readiness of so many people to contribute to the book launch, the publication of the book itself – could not be extricated from my terminal illness. This didn't daunt me. It gave me pleasure. I felt cherished, and even more importantly, I felt heard and understood.

The week before the launch, everything went according to plan – better than to plan, because by the time Avivah arrived, my second reprieve, my new chemo vacation, had given me enough time to regain some vital facets of normal life. I didn't need to sleep endlessly during the day. I could travel and walk around, and hold longish conversations. I could sit in a straight-backed chair for a couple of hours.

This was to be my third face-to-face meeting with Avivah in six years of weekly correspondence, and this time we would not just meet for one or two intense and memorable conversations, we would see each other frequently. Chooch had even arranged for the three of us to spend a few days at her brother-in-law's luxury beach house at a spectacular point on the Great Ocean Road. I was excited and anxious. I had no idea how our ever-increasing email intimacy would translate into real-life encounters. Over the years, we had become incredibly close, sharing both our Torah studies and many aspects of our lives. I was perhaps more forthcoming than she, but nonetheless I knew Avivah as well as I knew anyone, yet we'd had so little real-time experience with each other.

We met at the airport and fell into each other's arms. I needn't have worried. The email relationship slipped into a face-to-face intimacy without effort, without our needing to notice.

The book launch was scheduled a few days after Avivah arrived. It was to be held at the Centre for Jewish Civilization and would be followed by the first of her Melbourne lectures.

I generally find book launches, my own and others', inspiring but also embarrassing, and this launch was no exception. The inspiration came not from the book, but from the guests: my family, my friends, my students. And most of all, from my cancer. How could it not dominate? Everyone there knew my story. Death and creativity have always danced together in a way that has a power all its own.

Rachael was in Melbourne, and at the last minute, she and I decided to read duets from the book. I chose two poems that were written for two voices. We'd planned to read them at the end of the launch, but realized just as it was about to begin that she would need to leave early to catch her flight back to Sydney, and so we opened with them. There was no introduction, no greeting to silence the audience and get their attention; just our voices reading. It worked perfectly.

The speakers sang my praises. I smiled and blushed and looked at the floor. When

Avivah spoke, about the finding of a voice, I cried.

After the launch, Avivah's lecture. She spoke about the Matriarch Rachel as an "unknown woman" – a mystery to her husband Jacob and to her son Joseph. She described Rachel in Freudian terms, as Joseph's "dream navel" – the point in his dreams where the known touched the unknown. She took us to places of such depth that when she finished speaking, I felt as if I needed to swim back up to the surface. But I took my time. Being underwater with Avivah was not scary, it was blissful.

The following day, Avivah and Chooch and I set out for the beach house on the Great Ocean Road. It rained for the entire two days we were there, and that was perfect. We stayed indoors watching the wild ocean through huge picture windows and talked and cooked and ate and listened to music. For once, cancer took a back seat. I was still weak from the chemo, but my mind and my heart were engaged elsewhere, in Torah, in music, in friendship.

For those few days at the rainy beach house we stepped out of time. There was no schedule. The silences between us were as warm as the conversations. Like all good dreams, it had to end.

A few days later Doug, Avivah, and I were back at the airport, at the departure gate, saying goodbye.

Avivah and I opened our arms and hugged each other.

"*Nafshi l'nafshech*," she whispered into my ear. "My soul to your soul."

Ben. Was Ben here? Ben was here, reminding me.

The last words I heard him say.

"Why did you say that?" I asked Avivah.

"I don't know," she replied. She looked puzzled. "It's not an expression I use."

Soul to soul, our shadows roll, and I'll be with you when the deal goes down.

I suppose there are times in many people's lives when they feel the workings of something greater than themselves, when they are touched ever so gently as if by the brushing of a fluttering wing.

25

I still had two months to go before the next CT scan, and the results of that scan could mean the end of my chemo break, of my second reprieve, so I did my best to enjoy every day. I took my younger son Ben to a stage show, an adult send-up of *Sesame Street*. It was being staged at one of the oldest theaters in Melbourne, quite small and very ornate. At the interval, young men and women carrying trays of ice cream and chocolates walked up and down the aisles, just as they'd done when I was a child. Benny and I were in the front row. The show was hilarious. I was so proud of myself to have found something to share with my seventeen-year-old, sports-mad son. I wanted it to be a memory for both of us to cherish. That's really what I was doing. I was trying to create happy memories, writing the text as we lived it.

I took my daughter Orly to see *Sleeping Beauty* performed by the Australian Ballet. I'd been to the ballet once before, as a child with my grandmother. We saw Margot Fontaine and Rudolf Nureyev in *Swan Lake*. It's the most vivid happy memory of my childhood. Orly is an adult, but we were both enchanted by the sets and stunned by the beauty of the human body in motion.

Once, in a hypnotherapy session, Doris had conjured for me the image of a dancer being absolutely still. As Orly and I watched the princess fall into her deep sleep while the action continued on the other side of the stage, I examined the ballerina's "sleeping" body. Her toes remained pointed, slightly raised from the floor. Her limbs were exactly positioned. I could see her muscles and her ribs. Nothing moved. I could barely see her breathe. To do that must take years of practice and huge concentration.

I only managed to snare my older son for breakfast and a browse through some bookshops, but that's more his style, and we enjoyed ourselves. With my mother and my sister, on the other hand, I went to a fancy hotel on the Gold Coast for a couple of days. We had an entire apartment inside the hotel. By that time, the task of writing my story – this story – had become part of my daily routine. In the luxury hotel apartment I wrote at a desk facing the balcony, from which I could see mountains in the distance, rainforests at their feet, a small harbor with its nest of bobbing fishing boats, and an inlet leading out into the endless beach of crashing waves rolling in from an ocean that stretched to the horizon.

On the seashore of endless worlds, children play.

Both nights of our visit were blessed by a full moon, a blue moon. Before going to bed, I stood on the balcony and watched the moonlight fall upon the water, unwrapping itself like a swathe of luminescent silk across the ocean, from the horizon all the way to the inlet that was in line with our apartment. Never had I seen moonlight like that. I don't think I really knew the meaning of moonlight before those nights, even though it had always featured heavily in my teaching. I would speak about how the sun illuminates the surfaces of things and gives us a daytime world of high definition, a world of achievement, of progress, of goals. Moonlight, however, illuminates the world's soul. In moonlight, surfaces are obscured and we glimpse the heartland, a world in which there are no goals and nothing to achieve. Moonlight illuminates the innerness of things, and presents a world in which we can dream. When I saw the full moon laying out its carpet across the endless ocean, I understood what this meant.

My luck was holding. The scan showed no change. Stable! My chemo break was extended for another three months. Everyone was jubilant. My family cracked open some champagne and celebrated. I joined the general jubilance but in the back of my mind, familiar words echoed.

"There's no such thing as a body without a head."

The brain MRI was not due for another few months, and if I didn't have good results there, all this would become irrelevant. Nonetheless, I continued to enjoy my chemo-free vacation. I joined a gym and soon became hooked on daily exercise. After two years of cancer, I'd forgotten what it was like to work up a sweat, to feel the endorphins flowing, to return home beet-faced and energetic, for a shower and a salad lunch. A few more months of this and I'd be back to my old self – that would be my old, old self, the self that had thrived on daily exercise before work and study swallowed every waking minute.

I continued to teach my Thursday morning class. And I continued to write this memoir. I discovered that every episode I wrote about, I was somehow able to let go of. "Let go of" is not quite right. I was able to file away that part of my history, whereas before these episodes were jumping around inside me like random particles in the nucleus of an atom. As the file grew bigger, I became calmer and happier. Before each writing session, I read to myself, in a whisper, a poem by Rabindranath Tagore.

My song has put off her adornments. She has no pride of dress and decoration. Ornaments would mar our union; they would come between thee and me; their jingling would drown thy whispers.

My poet's vanity dies in shame before thy sight. O master poet, I have sat down at thy feet. Only let me make my life simple and straight, like a flute of reed for thee to fill with music.

I didn't want to "write." I wanted to allow what was inside of me to flow out of me. By the time I complete this writing I hope to be quite empty, and able to face whatever follows.

My only real physical annoyances during these months, apart from tiredness, were nightly headaches. They weren't acute, but still they worried me. I found myself counting the days until the brain MRI. The MRI loomed before me like a huge hurdle, blocking my view of the horizon. If it was clean, I'd be just about in remission. Perhaps the few remaining dots on my bones and lung would disappear, and I'd be officially in remission.

I'd promised myself that if that happened, I would stand at the *bimah* in our synagogue and recite the Thanksgiving Blessing, to be said by anyone who has survived a life-threatening situation. Often I sat with the women, listening to the service and dreaming of that moment. But usually I would interrupt my dream and spoil it. Why should I be saved when so many others aren't? How can there be a God in a world that is so unfair? How can God make sense in a world in which children die en masse and millions live and die in destitute misery?

And always, inexplicably, the same answer.

How can I not believe?

I don't think I was forcing belief in order to impose meaning on a chaotic world. My studies, and especially my intimacy with the writings of the Rabbi of the Warsaw Ghetto, had kind of hardwired me. Somewhere inside the chaos, inside the misery and the suffering, was God. Not distant, not a supreme director or master puppeteer, not separate at all.

Like the prophet Moses, the Rebbe of Piacezna heard God's voice inside the fire. I don't think he was deluding himself. He never withdrew into an ivory Torah tower to protect himself from the horrors of the Holocaust. He was utterly present every moment. He felt every blow, every wound, every death. And as the years wore on and the tortured ghetto groaned and collapsed around him, his writings grew stronger, more powerfully present, more painfully incisive. Shortly before he was taken, he wrote of the mystical concept of the hiding of God's face. When the world is lost in darkness, he wrote, God, as it were, hides His face, and retreats into what the *Zohar* calls His "crying rooms." But, wrote the Rebbe, this does not mean that He is inaccessible. He does not turn away from us. In our suffering, He is there with us. Sounds corny maybe, but I know that my most "spiritual" moments have also been my lowest moments. In my moments of suffering I acutely feel the presence of God. There are no atheists in foxholes, as they say. The Rebbe of Piacezna taught me that this is because God is right there with me in the foxhole.

When I first studied his teachings, I felt that the experiences of the Piacezna Rebbe were sacrosanct, that it would constitute some sort of travesty to apply them to my own petty vicissitudes. But the longer I stayed with him, the more this barrier dissolved.

I am only prepared to admit this to a nameless, faceless reader, for fear of being misunderstood. During that extended second reprieve, I admitted to myself that my years of cancer had been the most revelatory and transformative of my life. I could see myself and the world from a whole other, deeper perspective. Everything was illuminated by moonlight. I had insights that I doubt I would otherwise have had. Would I swap my insights for a longer life? Yes, I would, in a flash, but still it would be hard to surrender them, and return to a surface existence. This, I must stress, was an attitude adopted during a reprieve. When the roller coaster is racing downhill, when the cancer is active and I am broken by chemo, I am unaware of revelation and transformation. All I want is relief.

As the date for the MRI drew closer, the headaches increased in intensity. I wondered if they were due to anxiety, or to something more sinister. The wheels of my cancer began to grind, and I was hauled back into the fray. Before the riddle of the headaches was solved, I was forced to deal with other matters.

Lara had assured me that at age fifty-two, the recent rounds of chemo would put me into permanent menopause. When this was confirmed by a blood test, I was permitted to switch from the anti-hormonal Tamoxifen to Femara, a much weaker drug with fewer side effects and fewer risk factors. But a month after I began my chemo vacation, I began to bleed, heavily.

I was assured that I couldn't possibly be menstruating.

"It's just not possible," Lara said.

The not-possible revisited me the following month, then skipped a cycle just to keep us guessing, only to return with a vengeance the month after. I was sent to the gynecologist, who suggested a curette to rule out uterine cancer, which is one of the risk factors associated with Tamoxifen. More fear. More waiting. More worry.

The curette was a day procedure. I had a nightmarish awakening from the light general anesthetic, but it passed fairly quickly and an hour later I was returned to Doug, in the waiting room.

The results were clear. No uterine cancer, thank God, which led the doctors to conclude that the impossible had happened. My youthful body had bounced back after chemo, and after a corroborative blood test I was pronounced pre-menopausal again. I was very proud of my body. The body that had betrayed me was switching allegiances.

My body's resilience, however, meant that I'd either have to revert to Tamoxifen and suffer debilitating periods, or have my ovaries removed. I was strongly advised to opt for the latter. In view of the alternative, I had to agree.

The only free day for my gynecologist within the next month was the day for which my brain MRI had been scheduled. Nothing could be done about it. I had to postpone. I booked the next available MRI, which was three weeks later, at the end of the month.

The operation took place in a different hospital, even closer to my home. I was assured that this was a minor operation, keyhole surgery. I'd spend just one night in hospital. Once, this would have seemed like a big deal to me, another cause for anxiety, but I guess I was finally becoming a hardened old-timer. I really wasn't fazed about the prospect of having my ovaries removed. It didn't mean much more to me, physically and emotionally, than going to the dentist to have a tooth pulled. In a way, I was quite looking forward to it. I was going to a small private hospital which mostly catered to pregnant and birthing women. It had a reputation for good food and good care. I was looking forward to my upcoming overnight stay as a chance to be pampered.

When will I learn not to expect?

I checked in, accompanied by Doug, at 1 p.m., as expected. The operation was scheduled for 3 p.m.

After waiting twenty minutes or so, we were taken to a two-bed ward. Apparently the admission papers containing my request for a single room should have been mailed in advance, but I had handed them over when we arrived. There were no single rooms available, but the other occupant of my ward was only having a day procedure. So far, so good. It seemed I would have the room to myself for the night. I lay on my bed, and Doug pulled up a chair. The time dragged. An hour later a nurse appeared to tell us that the gynecologist had rushed off to an emergency call at St. Katherine's, and would be delayed for another hour or so. Okay. An hour passed, and another. Halfway through the next hour another nurse appeared with my hospital gown, cap and slippers, telling me to change into them. It seemed that my turn was approaching. Nope. Another hour passed. Doug had to leave. My roommate appeared. She seemed like a nice woman, but apart from telling me that she was here for an IUD, she wasn't interested in conversing. Finally, my turn arrived!

I was taken to a "holding bay" – yes, that's its name, written on a plaque on the wall. I was given a blanket and assured that the wait would not be long. The holding bay was a chair surrounded by drawn curtains that left me sitting in a space of about two leg spans. Outside the curtain, medical people came and went, chatting and joking. They couldn't see me. I was invisible. I waited and waited in the "holding bay," naked under my tied-in-the-back hospital gown, bald under my thin hospital cap. Why was I putting up with this? I had to act. I decided to count to fifty. When I got to fifty, I counted again. Then, without thinking, I grabbed the blanket, wrapped it around me and drew open the curtains. I was not going to be invisible! I paced the larger space, holding my head high, stopping to peer at diagrams and instructions pasted on the walls. Someone came in and asked me what I was doing.

"I'm not prepared to sit in there anymore," I replied, calmly.

My treatment at St. Katherine's had taught me that patients often have to be patient, but they never have to be victims. They never have to be humiliated.

My interrogator withdrew. My anesthetist, whom I had met earlier, came out and apologized. A little later, my gynecologist came, and also apologized. I accepted their apologies gracefully. It's all I'd wanted.

The operation was performed at 7:30 p.m. I'd had six hours to think about what was happening, which in retrospect I am grateful for. I had time to thank my ovaries for my children, the hearts of my heart, and to acknowledge the finality of what was happening.

The anesthetist found a vein and asked me a simple question. I got halfway through the answer.

Next thing I knew I was coming to in post-op. I felt like a dumb animal, shaking its head to and fro, trying to release itself from some kind of bondage. I couldn't make sense of myself or of anything around me. I begged to be taken back to Doug. Soon, they said, soon. When they wheeled me back to the ward, I was so relieved to see him, to feel my hand in his.

I recovered quickly from the surgery, but the memory of my restless awakening stayed with me. I never wanted to go through that again. I'd felt as if I'd lost myself, as if something in me had snapped and disconnected, and that parts of me were floating away, unanchored.

26

I was planning to wait another week or so before returning to the gym, to which I'd become completely addicted, as much for the high that the exercise gave me as for the sense of belonging in the real world, the world of the living, where middle-aged, middle-class Jewish women shopped and went to the gym and had coffee with friends.

But I would have to wait. After the oophorectomy – another new word to add to my growing medical lexicon – my nightly headaches grew worse, and began to extend into the day. Within a few weeks my head continually ached. At times I experienced sharp stabbing pains. The brain MRI was only a few weeks away. Perhaps the headaches were caused by anxiety. I tried to be stoic.

When the pain became overwhelming, I took Panadeine Fortes and soldiered on, until one Thursday morning, only days before the scan was scheduled. I was due to teach, but my head hurt so much I couldn't even think. I popped two Panadeine Fortes, and called Lara. The previous day I'd been walking in the street with two friends. We'd passed a busker, a young girl playing *You Are My Sunshine* on a trumpet. Despite the din, she made me smile, so I bent down to put some coins in her hat. When I straightened up again and tried to resume walking I felt as if someone had hit me from behind with a sledgehammer. I shrieked and doubled up in pain.

When I described the pain to Lara the following morning, she sounded worried. Fifteen minutes later, she called back. She couldn't get me an MRI at such short notice, but she'd booked me in for a CT scan at 11:30. I'd have to cut the class short and leave the house before my students.

The class went well. I spoke about the biblical account of the exodus from Egypt, about how God constantly interrupts the narrative, and the drama, to impress upon the Israelites the importance of the story that they are enacting. Like me with my children, God was creating memories. While the Israelites were still in Egypt, before the final plague, He was already giving instructions regarding future celebrations of the Passover festival, and commanding the Israelites to pass the story down from generation to generation.

The Haggadah, the text that sets out the order of the Passover Seder, instructs each of us, in every generation, to experience the liberation from slavery for him- or herself. The Haggadah tells the story of the journey from slavery to freedom, from sorrow to joy, from mourning to festivity, from darkness to great light in a way that enables one to experience redemption within the context of one's own life, one's own challenges.

We are brought out to tell the story, and through the telling we are brought out.

As I taught under the influence of all that codeine, I was flying high. The words were taking off, occasionally soaring, but my fear of the approaching brain scan remained heavy and intractable. It lurked in the shadows of my words. Was this the point? I wondered. Was all this happening just for the sake of the story? Would my story also be ultimately redemptive? Would I also be redeemed?

The Torah portion we were discussing begins with the final three plagues, collectively known as "the plagues of darkness." After Moses has proclaimed the final plague, the death of the firstborn, but before it devastates the land of Egypt, the narrative is interrupted once more. God commands the Israelites to count the months according to the lunar cycle. The Sages later interpreted this as a commandment to bless the new moon. According to Jewish law, sighting the new moon is a complicated business. At the end of its monthly cycle, the moon completely disappears and remains hidden for two days. In order to proclaim the new month, two witnesses had to peer into the moonless sky, into the black, black night, and wait for the fingernail of light to appear. The world was black, yet they looked and waited, knowing that this darkness was a prelude to great light.

Perhaps I too would be redeemed.

I rushed away with Doug after the class, leaving the students to chat over a cup of tea and lock the door behind them. The scan didn't take long. It was one of the shortest I could remember. I tried not to think about what this might imply. I tried to get on with the day. Sari, my GP friend, would hassle the hospital until she got the results and deliver them to me in person that evening, after work. We'd agreed upon this system months before, to save me the anxiety of waiting for a call. Sari is an exceptional friend. At times she worries about me more than I do myself. I know she goes through hell waiting for my results. During crises, she devotes many of her working hours to me, speaking to specialists, arranging appointments, home-delivering prescriptions.

This time, there was a slip-up. Sari received the results of my CT scan a few hours after it was taken, and immediately called Lara, who immediately secured me an appointment with a neurosurgeon. Before Sari had a chance to break the news to me, I received a call from Lara's receptionist.

"You'll be seeing Mr. Rodgers," she said. "You have an appointment for next Monday, 5 p.m., and your MRI will be Monday, 1 p.m."

I felt that familiar chill take hold of my body. "Who's Mr. Rodgers?"

The receptionist sounded testy. "He's a neurosurgeon."

A neurosurgeon? What? I asked to speak to Lara.

"She's not here," the receptionist barked.

"But, I don't understand."

Then she twigged. "Haven't you spoken to Lara?"

"No. No." I had also twigged. I hung up in a panic. What was happening? I pushed the words "brain surgery" away. I tried to shove them out of my mind, but they were too heavy. They wouldn't budge.

I heard my friend Susie's footsteps in the driveway. No. Not now. Not now.

She let herself in and found me clutching the phone, weeping.

"Don't speak!" I commanded. "Don't move! Not a word!"

Susie, usually so effusive, buttoned her mouth and dropped her parcels. She let them fall to the floor and stood stiff as a soldier outside Buckingham Palace while I raced around the house trying to reach Sari, Lara, God. Susie was a good friend to me that afternoon. She dropped her parcels. She must have been having all sorts of feelings, but she dumped none of them on me. I was very, very grateful.

Sari returned my call within minutes. She was devastated. She and Lara had agreed that she'd break the news to me and give me the details of the appointment with the neurosurgeon. Lara's receptionist had slipped up and called first, and dropped the bombshell.

"What is it?" I asked, as if I didn't know. "What's going on?"

"There's quite a bit of swelling over the left side of your cerebellum and some bleeding. The radiologist couldn't see what's causing it because the swelling's too extensive. Lara wants you to start taking Dexamethazone immediately. That will reduce the swelling and relieve the headaches. By Monday the swelling should be gone and an MRI will show us what's underneath."

"What could it be?" I mumbled, playing the idiot.

"It's some kind of mass. It could be necrosis, which is a kind of mass that can develop after radiation. Or it could be a tumor. Or it could be a bit of both."

I started taking Dexamethazone, a steroid, that afternoon. The relief was almost immediate. I was high as a kite, talking a mile a minute to anyone who would listen, but virtually pain-free.

The MRI confirmed that the two lesions in my cerebellum had grown, and that a new lesion had appeared much deeper in the brain tissue. I knew that this was not good news, but I took some comfort in learning that at least there were no other metastases elsewhere in my brain. And it was validating to know that I had not been imagining the massive headaches. Sounds petty, I know, but I'd so often accused myself of being a wuss, and I sometimes worried that others saw me as one. I think this fear dated back to primary school when I went crying to a teacher after falling onto the pavement and scraping my knee, only to be pushed aside and told that another girl had just broken her leg.

"Stop sniveling," I was told. "It's just a bit of blood. Can't you see that this girl here is seriously hurt?"

Deeply humiliated, I tried to stop sniveling as we waited for the ambulance.

I was almost proud to learn that my pain had been real enough to push some lesser mortal, someone who'd merely scraped her knee, out of the queue. For the time being,

I didn't ask for a detailed explanation of this latest diagnosis. I opted instead to take what little comfort I could find.

The neurosurgeon, Myron Rodgers, was as I would want a neurosurgeon to be: direct, steady, with well-shaped hands and fingers and decisive, powerful body language.

He cut to the point. No mercy. I'd been warned that he could be "overly direct."

"This operation is palliative, you know. It won't remove all the cancer from your brain."

I imagine him putting his feet up on his desk and crossing them when he said that, although I doubt that he did.

Once, I would have looked for a window to jump out of. Not any more. Ha! I thought. He can't scare me. I'm a seasoned cancer patient.

"Isn't all treatment for metastatic breast cancer palliative?" I asked, trying to look innocent, as if spurred on by an inquiring mind. "After all, I do have an incurable disease."

He grunted and almost smiled. I imagined him murmuring, *Touché*.

I felt very pleased with myself. Years ago, when I was first diagnosed, I would have been horrified if the word "palliative" was applied to me. Palliative meant you were dying. I couldn't hear of such a thing. Now I took it in my stride.

The brain surgeon described the operation, reiterating that as far as brain surgery went, it wasn't too complex. He'd remove as much as he could of the two tumors that had grown. The "palliative" meant that he couldn't remove them all. No, he wasn't saying that he *may* not remove them all. He definitely *could not* remove them all. If he did, I'd be seriously crippled. All he could do was take as much as possible, and thereby hopefully prolong my life for a limited amount of time. The new, deeper lesion was too difficult to reach by surgery. That would need stereotactic radiation, which I'd have after I'd recovered from the operation.

For all his brusque forthrightness, I liked him. He looked you straight in the eye and you could trust what he was saying.

I had just a few days to wait for the surgery, which was a blessing. I didn't want to think about it. Brain surgery had always been one of those things the thought of which made my bones go weak and sent chills down my spine. Cutting a hole in my skull and messing with my brain? No, better not to think about it.

I spent the few interim days sleeping, reading, and watching inane American sitcoms, one after another, until I felt cross-eyed.

Nonetheless, I couldn't hold back the creeping realization that had been triggered by the word "palliative." This would be a third attempt to knock out cancer cells in the same place in my brain. Somewhere in my reading, or perhaps in the eyes of my medical team, I'd picked up that this was most likely the end of the road for me.

I wasn't ready to think too much about this, not with the craniotomy looming. The human mind is a wonderful device. When overwhelmed, it seems to go into defense mode, refusing to admit that which threatens to overwhelm it. I had enough on my hands, or in my mind, dealing with the approaching surgery. Thoughts about why I needed it, and all that this implied, would have put me into overload.

It was only after the operation that I allowed the realization to surface. I'm not sure how I knew with such certainty. Perhaps it was that inbuilt knowing that Doris had taught me to access, or perhaps it was remembered from one of my illicit Google binges. Nonetheless, I wanted my certainty confirmed. And so I raised the issue with Sari my GP, with Lara my oncologist, with Dr. Birch my psychiatrist, even with a friend who happened to be a radio-oncologist. I was rather proud of my own cleverness, the tactics I used to get them to admit it.

"Don't worry," I'd say, "I know. I'm okay. I just want us to be open so we can discuss details."

When I said that, they'd stop squirming and feebly denying what we both knew to be true, and sadly nod their heads in confirmation. When they did that, it looked as if a weight was lifting from them. These were people who cared. And for me, each confirmation was a further jolt, another little stab, but it allowed my own realization to settle more easily in my conscious mind.

Strangely, my distress was not as great as I would have imagined, nor nearly as great as it was upon my first cancer diagnosis nearly three years earlier, nor as great as it was when I first heard that the cancer had spread to my brain.

I didn't feel defeated. I didn't feel inordinately terrified. Of course I wasn't over the moon with glee. I wanted to live, to survive, and I didn't discount that possibility. But I was surprised at how readily I accepted my survival for the small, the tiny, the minuscule possibility that it was.

The more I came to terms with these new developments, the more open I became with others, and the better I felt. For the first time in my life, my impending death rose into my conscious mind and I didn't push it away. I did eventually file it away, but only after I'd considered it thoroughly. I realized that I had something that many people were denied. I had a chance to accept the inevitability of my own death and to prepare myself, and others.

I realized that I needed to make a will. I thought that this would simply involve buying a standard form at the post office and filling it in, but the reality was much more complex. I needed to consult my brother the lawyer, the brother who had terrorized me as a child, the brother whom the years had mellowed, who had suffered, and softened, and with whom, after half a century on this earth, I had a loving relationship.

I could see that the prospect of advising me on this matter was terrifying for him. We needed to discuss various scenarios: if I died in three years, or two, or next year. And then we came to arrangements that would need to be put in place if I died this year. My youngest would still be in his final year of school. He would need a guardian. We needed to consider the household, how it would continue. When we came to that he hesitated. I urged him to remember that these were only hypotheticals. My will needed to be signed and sealed, but my death would never be disposed of so easily.

And then there was my mother. For a few weeks after the craniotomy, she and I avoided each other's eyes, unwilling to move together onto this new ground, until one afternoon at the hospital, we opened up.

I'd made an appointment to see Lara alone, without Doug, in order to induce a confirmation of my prognosis out of her. Our talk had been frank. We'd discussed palliative care and pain management. She'd agreed to start me on a new chemo combo that might possibly break through the blood-brain barrier. It hadn't been proven. No chemo had yet been proven to break through to the brain, but it was worth a try. So the end is never the end. We discussed side effects, what to do, how to cope. Suddenly, we were back in the world. I left with a fistful of prescriptions. When she was saying goodbye, Lara told me that she admired my attitude. Her eyes were glistening.

My mother had driven me to the meeting. On our way out we stopped at the pharmacy to drop in my prescriptions, and waited at the adjacent hospital café while they were being filled.

I turned to her. I hadn't planned this, but I knew it was about to happen.

"Mum," I said. "Do you know just how, um, serious my situation is?"

She looked at me, and for the first time since my initial diagnosis, her tough exterior crumpled.

"Yes," she said, and the tears began to flow. "I know. Oh my darling. My darling daughter." She began to sob. I put my arms around her. We were unused to these levels of intensity, but they must have always been there, floating between us, because nothing felt forced, nothing felt wrong.

"It's okay, Mum," I whispered. "If I compare myself to people in other places or to any other time in history, I've already lived a long time. And more than that, much more, I feel that I've achieved things. I don't feel like a failure."

Between sobs, my mother let out a hollow laugh. "Now *you're* comforting *me*."

"I should be comforting you. There's nothing more painful than the thought of losing a child, God forbid. I'm a mother too, you know."

And so we slowly eased ourselves back to more negotiable levels, but the moment of deep intimacy wasn't lost. She knew. I knew she knew. Everything had changed between us. I felt a great sense of relief. I hope she did also.

Time would move on, things would settle down. Perhaps we would all push what we all knew back into the recesses, and go back to planning a future. Yes, if things settled down, that's what would happen. That's the way it is. It's inevitable; it's human nature. We would settle back into life, until the next crisis took us and flung us back into the pit.

But I am way ahead of myself. I've gone beyond the end, to the weeks after the craniotomy, to opening up the prospect of death, and to new hopes pinned on unproven treatments.

The final verses of the Torah speak of what happened after the death of Moses. The sages ask: How can these verses be included, if they were written after the author's death?

A number of solutions to the conundrum are suggested, but my favorite is that of Rabbi Joshua. Up until these last few verses, he explains, Moses wrote the Torah in ink. After he died without ever reaching the Promised Land, he wrote in tears.

This is not a Torah and I, thank God, am no Moses. I am here, in the flesh, writing in ink of things that happened after the end. Perhaps I will still be here when you are reading of them. Perhaps I will not.

The craniotomy was for me an ending of sorts, and it is where I choose to conclude this memoir. Something happened then that opened up an ending; it made a hole great enough to birth the whole of God's creation. And in that ending is the beginning.

27

The week after the craniotomy was the first week, emerging from an amorphous mass of beginning. I remember on that first night, clinging to the bed-frame in intensive care, curled and fetal, feeling the explosion in my head, the act of creation. As the night wore on, I clung and curled, and the nurse let me be. I sensed the first separation, deep inside. After a few days I was aware of my two sides. One was familiar from before. I knew that side of me. It had a job to do, but now for the first time I felt that my job was done. And then there was this other me, a me I had never known, who presented a whole new task. At first I resisted. That's not mine, I said to myself. That belongs to someone else. It's not my job. Take it away from me. Give it to the person whose job it is.

By week's end I knew that we all have two tasks in life. Like Schrödinger's cat, two possibilities were equally real. Our tasks are to live, and to die. That job I had not wanted to take on, the job I wanted to assign to someone else, had existed since the beginning of time, way, way back, as far back as before my birth was my death. I didn't need to be afraid. This is just how the world works. We have our moment, and our moment is gone. But it is a good moment, forever significant, and it will never be erased. I am my moment in the history of the cosmos, and I am grateful for it.

Acknowledgments

I am deeply grateful to the Pratt Foundation and in particular to chief executive officer Sam Lipski for supporting this publication. Thanks also to the Australian Centre for Jewish Civilization for its involvement.

Many thanks to my agent Sharon Friedman, whose dedication and hard work have made this book a reality. Thanks also to Ilan Greenfield, Gefen's publisher, for sharing my vision. My friend and mentor Avivah Zornberg played a crucial role in steering the path of my manuscript, bringing it safely to a propitious home. Ita Olesker, Smadar Belilty, and Stuart Schnee of Gefen all deserve special mention.

Sandra Hogan in Queensland, Aviva Layton in Los Angeles, and Mark Baker and Melanie Landau in Melbourne were all instrumental in the editing process. Alex Skovron polished the final version until it shone.

I am also grateful to the family, friends, and medical professionals who have kindly allowed me to write about the points at which our lives have intersected.

And I am grateful to Doug for our enduring friendship.

Rabbi Kalonymus Kalmish Shapira, the holy Rebbe of Piacezna, wrote in his great book *Eish Kodesh* (Holy Fire) that even after a teacher has died, when students study his works his lips will move in the grave. Rabbi Shapira perished in the Holocaust, but he speaks to me frequently though the teachings in his text, and for this he has my everlasting thanks.